THE MYTH OF ADHD

AND OTHER LEARNING DISABILITIES

PARENTING WITHOUT RITALIN

by
Jan Strydom
and Susan du Plessis

Huntington House Publishers

Huntington House Publishers
P.O. Box 53788
Lafayette, Louisiana 70505

PRINTED IN THE UNITED STATES OF AMERICA

Library of Congress Card Catalog Number 00-108644
ISBN 1-56384-180-0

Scripture quotations are from the Holy Bible,
New International Version. Copyright 1973, 1978, 1984 by
International Bible Society.

Meet the Authors

This book is based on the research of Dr. Jan Strydom on learning and behavior problems over a period of more than twenty years. Dr. Strydom is a man of many talents. He holds a doctorate in education and an M.A. in philosophy, speaks several languages, is a trained opera singer and is internationally recognized as a chess problem composer. He is a father of three and grandfather of two.

Susan du Plessis has been co-researcher of Dr. Strydom for more than ten years. She holds B.Div. and an honors degree in psychology. She is author of three books, among others *The Truth about Learning Disabilities* (1994) and its complete revision, *The New Truth about Learning Disabilities* (1997). Susan and her husband, Henk, have two sons.

Content

Foreword
by Dr. Jan Strydom

This is a book for parents who desire the best for the future of their children. Parents are at present floundering around in the quagmire of contradictory ideas that they are being fed by the so-called "experts" on child rearing. In the process, parents become increasingly ignorant. In fact, there has probably never been a time in the history of the world when there has been more mind-boggling ignorance on children than there is now. The result is that an activity that should be one of the most enjoyable and fulfilling in the life of any person—raising one's children—has for many been turned into a nightmare. A further result is that children have probably never suffered more than they do now.

A shocking example of this suffering was described in the morning newspaper a few weeks ago in a report of a young schoolboy on the threshold of his adult life, who committed suicide by shooting himself. In the same newspaper appeared a separate article listing the names of several other children who had recently killed themselves. A psychiatrist, in response to a question about the causes of such tragedies, stated that it was mere coincidence that prompts so many children to commit suicide.

Such a response is typical of the superficial thinking that prevails in our times. The psychiatrist's response strongly supports my expectation that, in times to come, the present age will be referred to as the Age of Superficiality.

As this book shockingly and clearly indicates, suicide is but one of many child and youth problems that abound at present. Not only are there the problems of attention, reading, and math that so alarmingly affect children's ability to perform adequately at school, but also the even-more-alarming incidences of youth suicide, criminal activity, and drug abuse.

This book stresses a point that is apparently universally over-looked. How can one hope to solve any problem without knowing its cause? Many of the experts who involve themselves with youth problems seem to believe that "the clinical need for appropriate treatment"[1] is far more pressing than the identification of causes.

Those who do concern themselves with causes seem to be inclined to compartmentalize. For example, when confronted by the attention and learning difficulties of children, these experts look for "disabilities," "disorders," "dysfunctions," and "syndromes," apparently believing that these are all indicative of something being "wrong" in the brain of the child. The suicides, as stated above, are attributed to such nebulous vagaries as "coincidence," whereas the violence on TV is accused of being the cause of the violent criminality in present-day youth.

This book attempts to take a more comprehensive view of the matter. Authors, however, who attempt to avoid the superficial think-ing that typifies our present age unfortunately often find that they thereby expose themselves to personal attack, as was experienced by Richard Milton, the author of one of the references in this book, *The Facts of Life: Shattering the Myths of Darwinism*. In a later edition, Milton writes that, in a review of the book, Richard Dawkins, reader in zoology at Oxford university, "devoted two thirds of his review to attacking my hardback publishers, Fourth Estate, for their irrespon-sibility in daring to accept a book criticizing Darwinism, and the remainder to assassinating my own character."[2]

This reaction to Milton's book indicates that there are three parts to the present human dilemma. One is the betrayal of the human spirit, the assertion of dogma that closes the mind.

Recently, my wife and I had dinner with two friends in a res-taurant. A few days before this dinner, the woman had just com-pleted a thesis for a Master's degree in education. She talked very excitedly about everything she had learned in the course of her research and studies. At one stage, she asked the waiter for a glass of water. When it arrived, she put it in the middle of the table.

"If I look at this glass of water from where I sit, I see certain things. You [pointing at me] look at it from where you sit and see something else. He [her husband] looks at it from where he sits, and sees something else again, as does she [meaning my wife]." She was hinting at Thomas Kuhn's ideas, of course. The thought that came to my mind immediately, however, was that she was unknowingly expressing one of the most serious problems of our times. Many people are inclined to jump to conclusions after looking at a problem from just one perspective and then make dogmatic claims about it.

Bronowski (with my italics) has an interesting example to warn us against such unwise practices:

> Think of the puzzles that the electron was setting . . . The quip among professors was . . . that on Mondays, Wednesdays, and Fridays the electron would behave like a particle; on Tuesdays, Thursdays, and Saturdays it would behave like a wave. . . . That is what the speculation and argument was about. And that requires, not calculation, but insight, imagination—if you like, metaphysics. I remember a phrase that Max Born used. . . . He said: "I am now convinced that theoretical physics is actual philosophy."
>
> Max Born meant that the new ideas in physics amount to a different view of reality. The world is not a fixed, solid array of objects, for it cannot be fully separated from *our perception* of it. It shifts under our gaze, it interacts with us, and the knowledge that it yields *has to be interpreted by us*.[3]

The trouble is that there are people who seem to be satisfied with *any* interpretation, or, as Popkin and Stroll expressed it, "There are always people who are ready to accept almost any view."[4] That explains why it is so, as the same two authors remark, that the "history of science is replete with theories that have been thoroughly believed by the wisest men and were then thoroughly discredited."[5] It also explains how ideas like ADHD (et cetera) could have become so widely accepted. In fact, no theory or belief has ever been so absurd that there has not been someone who believed it and argued for it. Throughout the course of history, people have also attempted to impose their beliefs on others—often even the most outlandish and obviously ridiculous beliefs—and have tried to punish those who rejected them. The early Greek philosopher, Anaxagoras, for example, was exiled from Athens for saying that the moon was a stone. Galileo, as is well known, was interrogated by the Inquisition and forced to recant on pain of being burned at the stake. Today, "rebel" scientists, those who do not go along with the "popular" views of the "orthodox scientists," are not punished by physical exile, but by attempts to prevent them from getting their views published; nor by being physically burned at the stake, but by attempts to present them as ridiculous or having their characters assassinated.

Two is the belief that the end justifies the means. Bronowski tells a horrifying story to illustrate this:

> [Szilard] wanted to keep the patent secret. He wanted to prevent science from being misused. And, in fact, he assigned the patent to the British Admiralty, so that it was not published until after the war.
>
> But meanwhile war was becoming more and more threatening. . . . Early in 1939 Szilard wrote to Joliot Curie asking him if one could make a prohibition on publication. He tried to get Fermi not to publish. But finally, in August of 1939, he wrote a letter which Einstein signed and sent to President Roosevelt, saying (roughly), "Nuclear energy is here. War is inevitable. It is for the President to decide what scientists should do about it."
>
> But Szilard did not stop. When in 1945 the European war had been won, and he realized that the bomb was now about to be made and used on the Japanese, Szilard marshalled protest everywhere he could. He wrote memorandum after memorandum. One memorandum to President Roosevelt only failed because Roosevelt died during the very days that Szilard was transmitting it to him. Always Szilard wanted the bomb to be tested openly before the Japanese and an international audience, so that the Japanese should know its power and should surrender before people died.
>
> As you know, Szilard failed. . . . The first atomic bomb was dropped on Hiroshima in Japan on 6 August 1945 at 8:15 in the morning. I had not been long back from Hiroshima when I heard someone say, in Szilard's presence, that it was the tragedy of scientists that their discoveries were used for destruction. Szilard replied, as he more than anyone else had the right to reply, that it was not the tragedy of scientists: "it is the tragedy of mankind."[6]

It is at present the tragedy of mankind that people, who profess to be "scientists"—the inventors of "ADHD," "hyperactivity," "oppositional defiant disorder," "conduct disorder," "Tourette syndrome," "learning disabilities," and all other "syndromes," "dysfunctions" and "disorders" of that ilk—are working very hard toward the destruction of children.

The tragedy these people have brought into our world and into millions of lives already far outweighs that brought about by the atomic bomb. I hope this book will be more successful than Szilard's efforts were. I hope it will at least be a small step towards counteracting the giant leap of unnecessary tragedy that has been brought upon our world.

Three is the fact that history tends to repeat itself. Van der Westhuizen indicates that not only is there linearity in history, but also cyclicity.[7] Both, of course, have their fortunate and unfortunate aspects.

One of the fortunate aspects of the fact that there is a linear continuation in history means that people like the coauthor of this book and me, who wish that ideas like ADHD and the others discussed in this book will soon go away, are going to get our wish. Intellectual movements that land at the top of the academic pecking order will inexorably be deposed again.

On the other hand the unfortunate aspect is, of course, that in the meantime, until sense starts to prevail again, millions of children have to suffer unnecessarily.

The most unfortunate aspect of the cyclicity is that inevitably sometime in the future similar nonsensical ideas will arise again, just as present misconceptions are repetitions of previous occurrences of science taking a wrong track. Lavine has indicated that

> Many people in our contemporary world are very close to the Sophists in their beliefs. Like the Sophists, they are skeptics, doubtful of any claims to knowledge, especially when authorities are in conflict and fight among themselves—for example, about how to teach children to read.[8]

The problem about contemporary scientific research is that it is no longer based on achievements,[9] but on speculation. That is why the creators of ADHD, as they are identified in this book, have to explain away their failures by asserting that ADHD—and all the other problems of children that prevail at present—are "incurable." The research described in this book, which is emphatically *not* based on speculation but on achievement, clearly exposes the absurdity of such a claim.

For that reason it is of the utmost importance that all parents *must* read this book. No parent can afford to continue subjecting his or her child to the destruction that inevitably follows the ideas of the creators of ADHD. The time has come for parents to become more discriminating consumers when it comes to accepting advice on what to do with their children. Please, parents, when a so-called "expert" tells you that his own child also suffers from ADHD, immediately grab your child and run as far away from such a person as you possibly can; he has nothing to say to you. If he cannot solve the problems of his own child, what can he possibly do for yours? If he tells you that your child will "suffer" from this "condition" for life, get up and run. He has nothing to offer you or your child.

Never in history have parents been more in need of sensible advice, advice that *works*, advice that definitely *succeeds* in giving their children a *life of better quality*. That is the kind of advice they will find in this book.

Notes:

1. Lloyd, J. W., "A Commentary on Learning Disabilities," in *Learning Disabilities: Nature, Theory and Treatment*, N. N. Singh & I. L. Beale (eds.), (New York: Springer Verlag, 1992), 575.

2. Milton, R., *The Facts of Life: Shattering the Myths of Darwinism* (London: Corgi Books, 1993), 9.

3. Bronowski, J., *The Ascent of Man* (London: Macdonald Futura Publishers, 1981), 229.

4. Popkin, R. H., & Stroll, A., *Philosophy Made Simple* (London: W. H. Allen, 1969), xviii.

5. Ibid., 167.

6. Bronowski, *The Ascent of Man*, 233-234.

7. Van der Westhuizen, H. G., *Vertrou op God* (Pretoria: HAUM, 1977), 2.

8. Lavine, T. Z., *From Socrates to Sartre: The Philosophic Quest* (New York: Bantam Books, 1984), 25.

9. Cf. Mouton, J., & Marais, H. C., *Metodologie van die Geesteswetenskappe: Basiese Begrippe* (Pretoria: RGN, 1989), 146.

1.

A Frog in a Pot

"Stefano always has the last say in any argument," says his mother. "I think he will probably become a lawyer one day."

Stefano, seven, is a bright little boy who learned to read, write, and understand math way ahead of other children. His parents took him out of preschool because the curriculum wasn't challenging enough.

But Stefano has his problems—he bites, screams, fights, and can't fit in with other children at a "normal" school. Stefano has been diagnosed as suffering from "Attention Deficit Hyperactivity Disorder." Since he was 4-years-old, he has been taking the drugs Ritalin and Catapress to treat its symptoms.

"He is sociable and has sports skills, but when his behavior kicks in, people just see him as naughty," says his mother.

Because he couldn't "fit in," Stefano was forced to go to three different schools before reaching first grade. Eventually he had to be taken out of mainstream schools because teachers and students couldn't cope with him. Stefano now attends a special school.[1]

Although "attention deficit hyperactivity disorder" (ADHD) has been a buzz word for a number of years, there is still little agreement as to what it is, what causes it, and how it should be treated. While its advocates claim it to be a mental disease which some say afflicts up to 20 percent of the population, its opponents deny its very existence. Their argument is that the behavior characteristics associated with this disorder—a short attention span, poor concentration, daydreaming, hyperactivity, impulsiveness and disruptive behavior—are normal of childhood. Consider Tom Sawyer's indifference to schooling and Huckleberry Finn's "oppositional" behavior, they would say. Were they normal or suffering from ADHD?

Another point frequently made by the opponents of ADHD is that this disorder has no definite symptoms. How dreamy is too dreamy? Where is the line between an energetic child and a hyperactive one, between a spirited, risk-taking kid and an alarmingly impulsive one, between flexibility and distractibility?

While some are praising Ritalin, the most popular treatment for ADHD, others are disclaiming it:

> There is something odd, if not downright ironic, about the picture of millions of schoolchildren filing out of "drug-awareness" classes to line up in the school nurse's office for their midday dose of amphetamine. It is this sort of image that fires the imaginations of Ritalin's critics—critics like child psychiatrist Carl L. Kline of the University of British Columbia who was reported as saying that "Ritalin is nothing more than a street drug being administered to cover the fact that we don't know what's going on with these children."[2]

"I would gladly take my kids off the drugs if someone would give me something else that works. We've tried the alternative treatments—diets, the whole bit," said Opal Flanagan, a mother whose two teenaged sons have been diagnosed with ADHD and have taken a wide variety of drugs during the past decade. She herself was diagnosed with ADHD in 1992.

Mrs. Flanagan's youngest son is fifteen and was diagnosed at age five. "We knew he had some speech problems at four when he was in preschool. Then later he had trouble concentrating, would not sit still. We had him tested. We were told he had ADHD." Her son took Ritalin for eight years. He was switched to Dexedrine, another stimulant, two years ago. In addition to Dexedrine, he also takes Tegretol and Imipramine for bipolar disorder and manic depression, respectively.

Her oldest son is sixteen and was diagnosed with ADHD at eight. "We didn't see it in him because he wasn't hyperactive," Mrs. Flanagan said. "His grades dropped from *A's* to *C, D,* and *F.* But within three weeks of getting Ritalin, he was a success again. On the first day of third grade, he came to me and said he stayed focused."[3]

Erin's parents would probably agree with Mrs. Flanagan. They would also take their child off Ritalin if there were something else that could "do the job." In fact, last spring they enrolled her at a center that uses behavior modification to control the symptoms

related to ADHD. She attended the school's summer program.
"It was a horrid summer," Erin's father recalls:

> Behavior modification was controlling a lot of things, but
> the impulsivity would snowball. She would be told not to
> touch something—whether a car's gearshift or a radio or a
> computer. You'd say "Don't touch," and she would look at
> you and you could see she heard, but you'd see her hand
> slowly moving toward it—and she knew if she touched it,
> she would have to take time out or lose her TV privileges—
> but she would touch it anyway. And when the consequences
> happened, she would have an hour-long temper tantrum. It
> made for a no-fun life.[4]

Whether one chooses to accept or to deny the ADHD label,
sing the praises of or reject stimulants such as Ritalin, the fact
remains that worldwide there are millions of parents and teachers
who find themselves on a "daily battleground" with children.[5] These
children are uncontrollable to a lesser or greater extent—hyperactive, impulsive, aggressive, loners, destructive at times, with adjustment, behavioral, learning, and socialization problems.

There is no question that ADHD can disrupt lives. Kids with
this "disorder" frequently have few friends. Their parents may be
ostracized by neighbors and relatives who blame them for failing to
control their children. "When you're out in public, you're always on
guard," one mother said. "Whenever I'd hear a child cry, I'd turn to
see if it was because of Jeremy."[6]

They are also prone to accidents, says neurologist Roseman.
"These are the kids I'm going to see in the emergency room this
summer. They rode their bicycles right into the street and didn't
look. They jumped off the deck and forgot it was high."[7]

Distressed neighbors and broken bones, however, are hardly the
full picture. ADHD is often accompanied by learning problems, as
well as behavioral and emotional problems. Coordination problems
are often encountered, and up to 60 percent have some dysfunction
of early speech development. Although these children usually acquire speech at the appropriate stage in the first year of life, they
tend to be late in further extending and developing their expressive
language.[8] Eighty percent of children with ADHD have problems
with reading, spelling, and writing, and 60 to 70 percent will become aggressive or develop behavior problems.[9]

Children with ADHD suffer to a significant degree from a low self-esteem. As a result of their poor self-esteem, these children employ various techniques to gain acceptance by their peer group. For this reason, they are much more easily influenced and led by other children, and are frequently exploited.[10]

Twenty to 30 percent of children with ADHD experience anxiety disorders and up to 75 percent experience depression.[11] Children with ADHD often have poor sleeping habits; 30 percent suffer from bed-wetting, and 15 percent from encopresis.[12]

If any one hundred children with ADHD are followed from birth to adulthood, by ages five to seven, half to two-thirds will be hostile and defiant, a condition psychiatrists call "oppositional defiant disorder" (ODD).[13] Symptoms associated with ODD include the following: often loses temper; often argues with adults; often actively defies or refuses to comply with adults' requests or rules; often deliberately annoys people; often blames others for his or her mistakes or misbehavior; is often touchy or easily annoyed by others; is often angry and resentful; and is often spiteful and vindictive.

By ages ten to twelve, this group will start running the risk of developing what psychiatrists call "conduct disorder" (CD)[14]—consistent lying, stealing, running away from home or regular truancy from school. Other symptoms include mugging or armed robbery, deliberate fire-setting, sexual molestation or even rape, and physical cruelty to animals or people. Eventually, 20 to 40 percent of children with ADHD will develop CD.[15] Szatmari et al. found that ADHD males are fourteen times, and ADHD females are forty times more likely to develop CD than "normal" children are.[16]

By the time this group of one hundred reaches sixteen, approximately 75 percent will continue to have problems at school, with their families, or with authorities. As teens, the ADHD group may exercise poor judgment when they are unsupervised and with peers.[17] Particularly those with childhood ODD are at much higher risk of early substance abuse (25-30 percent) and social rejection (50 percent or more).[18]

School can be a shattering experience for these children. Frequently reprimanded and turned out, they lose any sense of self-worth and fall ever further behind in their work. Almost 60 percent can be anticipated to have failed one grade in school;[19] about a third fail to graduate from high school.[20] They also experience high rates of suspension and expulsion from school.[21]

If we were to follow the same set of individuals even further forward in time, a surprising prevalence of problems would yet be found. As adults, as many as 50 to 65 percent would still be symptomatic for ADHD.[22] Approximately 50 percent of those with CD will develop into antisocial adults (previously they were called psychopaths). Of the group of conduct-disordered children who do not develop into antisocial adults, a high percentage will have other psychiatric problems, including drug and alcohol abuse. They are likely to have more psychiatric hospitalizations, be unemployed or underemployed, and to have impaired marital and family relationships with more frequent divorces and remarriages. They also tend to have higher arrest rates for drunken driving and criminal acts. One in ten children with ADHD turn out to be severely dysfunctional adults and may require hospitalization or even end up in jail.[23]

According to research by Hawkins,[24] Thornberry,[25] Martinez and Bournival,[26] and Matazow and Hynd,[27] the correlation between ADHD and antisocial behavior is so high that ADHD can be considered as a predisposing risk factor. According to Baker, as many as 90 percent of those in jail currently have hyperactivity, and over 60 percent could have full-blown ADHD[28]—a significant percentage, considering that 3 to 5 percent of the population is generally said to have ADHD.

It is an article of faith among ADHD researchers that the right interventions can prevent such dreadful outcomes. "If you can have an impact with these kids, you can change whether they go to jail or to Harvard Law School," says psychologist James Swanson at the University of California.[29] And yet, despite decades of research, no one is certain exactly what the optimal intervention should be.

The problem is that successful intervention is dependent on finding the *cause* of a problem. Most problems can only be solved if one knows what *causes* that particular problem. A disease such as scurvy claimed the lives of thousands of seamen during their long sea voyages. The disease was cured fairly quickly once the *cause* was discovered, viz. a Vitamin C deficiency. A viable point of departure in this case would thus be to ask the question, "What is the *cause* of ADHD?"

In 1932, Frankwood E. Williams, the director of the U.S. National Committee for Mental Hygiene, reflecting over the past two decades of psychiatry, confessed, "The basic question with which psychiatrists and particularly those interested in mental hygiene start is—What are the causes of mental and nervous disease? This question has been repeatedly raised during the twenty-two years of organized mental hygiene until it has almost become a ritual and like a ritual has led to nothing except repetition—not even a start."[30] In 1995, Dr. Rex Cowdry, then-director of the U.S. National Institute of Mental Health (NIMH) underlined Williams' words with the confession: "We do not know the causes." And, because psychiatry does not know the causes of mental disease, he also had to admit: "We don't have methods of 'curing' these illnesses yet."[31]

What the reader is bound to discover in this book is that psychiatry, and its cousin psychology, the very two disciplines working so hard to try and find biological causes of so-called mental diseases, *have in fact caused many of these "mental diseases."* This is particularly true of ADHD.

Such a suggestion may come as a shock to most readers. However, no other avenue of research has so far lead to any reasonable explanation for the causes of the myriad of child problems that plague our present society. No form of intervention or treatment has delivered any significant results. If the reader will approach the above suggestion with an open mind, and will continue to follow the arguments as set out in the ensuing pages, he will undoubtedly find that not only are the arguments logical, but they lead to unprecedented practical results.

A brief allegorical interlude should enable the reader to gain an understanding of the way in which the whole world has been hoodwinked over the past few decades and lulled into a false acceptance of the idea that mysterious "disorders," "dysfunctions," and "syndromes" are at work in the brains and minds of our children. What has been happening to us over the past few decades can be compared to the situation of a frog in a pot of cold water on a stove. If the stove is switched on so that the water will very gradually become warmer and warmer, the frog will remain oblivious to the danger that awaits him. If somebody should suggest to the frog that he will cook to death in a few minutes, he will scoff at the idea. He will only realize the danger when it is too late. It is to be hoped that this book does not come too late or that its message will not be taken seriously only when it is too late.

To fully understand how psychology and psychiatry have caused ADHD and many of the other "syndromes" and "disorders" which our children today supposedly suffer from, it is necessary to take note of the influence they have had on the thought of Western society—especially on child education. Many of these ideas have started in North America, from whence they have engulfed the rest of the Western world and have recently also found their way into many non-Western countries. As the reader will discover, the effects of these ideas have been destructive in the extreme and have in essence created the mental diseases which children are today diagnosed with, as well as many of the other problems our children are struggling with. Indeed, it could well be stated that there has never been a time in the history of the world when children have had as many problems as they have today.

Criticism against psychiatry and psychology is not unusual. As a matter of fact, the most outspoken critics against these two disciplines are people who are inside these professions. One such person is Dr. Thomas Szasz, Professor Emeritus of Psychiatry at the State University of New York at Syracuse, Lifetime Fellow of the American Psychiatry Association, and author of twenty-three books—inter alia the classic *The Myth of Mental Illness*. He unequivocally stated that "child psychology and child psychiatry cannot be reformed. They must be abolished."[32]

The difference, however, between this book and many others who blame psychiatry and psychology for creating "problem children," is that this book does not only criticize, but also offers a viable solution. Knowing the cause of a problem, in most cases, is only the first step in solving that particular problem. If, for example, your car breaks down and you know that the accelerator is the cause of the breakdown, this knowledge alone will not fix the car. You will have to know *a lot more* about cars to get your car back on the road again. In the same way, knowing that psychiatry and psychology have brought ADHD into being will not solve the problem. Before we shall be able to help our children to overcome their problems with concentration, emotions, behavior, and learning, we shall have to know *a lot more* about people in general. And, we shall have to know *even more* about children in particular.

Notes

1. Kambouropoulos, K., " 'Be wary' on hyper young," *Progress Press*, 17 August 1998, 6.

2. Livingston, K., "Ritalin: Miracle drug or cop-out?" *The Public Interest*, vol. 127, 15 April 1997.

3. Hadnot, I. J., "A prescription for controversy," *The Dallas Morning*, 24 February 1997.

4. Gibbs, N., "The age of Ritalin," *Time,* 30 November 1998.

5. Doyle, C., "Options for the 'hyper child,'" *Woman's Weekly to the Natal Mercury,* 27 February 1992, 8.

6. Wallis, C., "Behavior: Life in overdrive," *Time,* 18 July 1994, 42.

7. Ibid.

8. Serfontein, G., *The Hidden Handicap* (Sydney: Simon & Schuster, 1990), 47.

9. Wolfish, M. G., "Attention deficit disorder (the hyperactive child)," *Modern Medicine of South Africa,* November 1988.

10. Serfontein, G., *The Hidden Handicap,* 56-57.

11. McKinney, J., Montague, M., & Hocutt, A., "A synthesis of the research literature on the assessment and identification of attention deficit disorder," *Education of Children with Attention Deficit Disorder* (Washington, DC: U.S. Department of Education, 1993), 96; Dykman, R., Ackerman, P., & Raney, T., *Assessment and Characteristics of Children with Attention Deficit Disorder* (Washington, DC: U.S. Department of Education, 1993).

12. Wolfish, "Attention deficit disorder (the hyperactive child)."

13. Goldstein, S., & Goldstein, M., *Hyperactivity: Why Won't My Child Pay Attention?* (New York: John Wiley & Sons, Inc., 1992); Barkley, R. A., cited in A. Martinez & B. Bournival, "ADHD: The tip of the iceberg?" *The ADHD Report,* vol. 3(6), 1996, 5-6.

14. Wallis, "Behavior: Life in overdrive."

15. Goldstein & Goldstein, *Hyperactivity: Why Won't My Child Pay Attention?;* Barkley, cited in Martinez & Bournival, "ADHD: The tip of the iceberg?"

16. Szatmari, P., Boyle, M., & Offord, D. R., "ADHD and conduct disorder: Degree of diagnostic overlap and differences among correlates," *Journal of the American Academy of Child and Adolescence Psychiatry,* vol. 28(6), 1989, 865-872.

17. Wodrich, D. L., *Attention Deficit Hyperactivity Disorder: What Every Parent Wants to Know* (Baltimore: Paul H. Brookes Publishing Co., 1994), 23.

18. Barkley, R. A., "ADHD, Ritalin, and conspiracies: Talking back to Peter Breggin," Russell Barkley Book Review, CH.A.A.D., www.catalog.com/chadd/news/Russ-review.htm.

19. Wodrich, *Attention Deficit Hyperactivity Disorder,* 23.

20. Wallis, "Behavior: Life in overdrive."

21. McKinney, Montague & Hocutt, "A synthesis of the research literature on the assessment and identification of attention deficit disorder."

22. Wodrich, *Attention Deficit Hyperactivity Disorder,* 23.

23. Weisberg, L. W., & Greenberg, M. D., *When Acting Out Isn't Acting* (New York: Bantam Books, 1991), 120, 123.

24. Hawkins, J., "Controlling crime before it happens: Risk-focused prevention," *National Institute of Justice Journal,* vol. 229, 1995.

25. Thornberry, T., "Risk factors for youth violence," in L. McCart (ed.), *Kids and Violence* (Washington, DC: National Governors Association, 1994).

26. Martinez & Bournival, "ADHD: The tip of the iceberg?"

27. Matazow, G., & Hynd, G., "Right hemisphere deficit syndrome: Similarities with subtypes of children with attention deficit disorder," Paper prepared at the Annual Convention of the International Neuropsychological Society, San Diego, CA.

28. Baker, D., "Identifying probationers with ADHD-related behaviors," *Criminal Justice and Behavior,* vol. 22, 1995.

29. Wallis, "Behavior: Life in overdrive."

30. "Witch doctors, shamans. The birth of the 'cult' of child psychology," *Psychiatry: Betraying and Drugging Children* (Los Angeles: CCHR, 1998), 8-11.

31. Ibid.

32. "Psychiatry destroys futures," *Psychiatry Manipulating Creativity* (Los Angeles: CCHR, 1997), 46-49.

2.

The Myth of ADHD

In 1851, a Louisiana physician and American Medical Association member, Samuel A. Cartwright, published a paper in the *New Orleans Medical and Surgical Journal* in which he described a new medical disorder he had recently identified. He called it drapetomania, from *drapeto,* meaning to flee, and *mania,* an obsession. He used this term to refer to a condition that he felt was prevalent in runaway slaves. Dr. Cartwright felt that with "proper medical advice, strictly followed, this troublesome practice that many Negroes have of running away can be almost entirely prevented."[1]

If Dr. Cartwright would submit his paper today, even to the most unrespectable medical journal, it would merely raise a laugh, or Dr. Cartwright himself would be considered disordered. But in 1851, slavery was still acceptable and therefore his invented disorder was not frowned upon.

Diseases—both physical and mental—are as old as mankind itself. However, they are not universal. As Ivan Illich wrote, "each civilization defines its own diseases. What is sickness in one might be chromosomal abnormality, crime, holiness, or sin in another. For the same symptom of compulsive stealing [in different communities] one might be executed, tortured to death, exiled, hospitalized or given alms or tax money."[2]

The definition of disorders may also differ from one generation to the next. A specific behavior that one generation considers abnormal, another generation may interpret as quite normal. Not too long ago homosexuality was considered a mental illness. It no longer is.

On the other hand, there are numerous aspects of human behavior which were considered normal twenty years ago but are today defined by psychiatry as syndromes, disorders, or disabilities. Under the heading, "Don't stop the insanity (my therapist needs the money)," Mark Syverud, editor of *The Daily Messenger,* comments in a tongue-in-cheek manner on the untenability of this kind of diagnostic practice:

> Beware, a new book shows that an epidemic of mental illness is sweeping the nation. Does your 10-year-old dislike doing her math homework? Better get her to the nearest couch because she's got No. 315.4, *Developmental Arithmetic Disorder.* Maybe you're a teenager who argues with his parents. Uh-oh. Better get some medication pronto because you've got No. 313.8, *Oppositional Defiant Disorder.*
>
> And if your wife won't tell you that she snuck out to the outlet mall last Saturday, then she's definitely got 313.2, *Selective Mutism.* Omigosh! My family is full of psychos. Trust me, I'm not making these things up. (That would be *Fictitious Disorder Syndrome.*) . . .
>
> Only a decade ago, psychiatrists said one in 10 Americans had a mental illness. Now, according to the manual, half the population is mentally ill. How the other half stays sane remains a mystery. The manual will have to be updated annually because mental health professionals and defense lawyers keep discovering new illnesses. Just since the beginning of the year the experts have unearthed these new disorders:
>
> Lottery Stress Disorder (or LSD): A London psychiatrist discovered the outbreak among losers who experienced "definition of mood and feelings of hopelessness" when their numbers didn't come in.
>
> Chronic Tax Anxiety Syndrome (CTAS): A Washington psychotherapist specializes in treating couples who suffer from excessive worry, sleeplessness and marital squabbling every April. . . .
>
> I know there are some cynics out there who will scoff at these new diagnoses. Maybe you think it's all psychobabble, just a gimmick to make money for the therapists. You wouldn't be caught dead on a psychiatrist's couch.
>
> You people are in serious denial. As a matter of fact, your unwillingness to seek professional help is itself a symptom of a serious mental problem. It's right here in the book: 15.81 *Noncompliance with Treatment Disorder.*[3]

The book or manual Mark Syverud is referring to is the *Diagnostic and Statistical Manual* (DSM), the bible of psychiatrists, psychologists and related specialists. The DSM is a catalogue, created by the American Psychiatric Association (APA), listing all the mental disorders with their various criteria that mankind can supposedly suffer from.

After the first DSM was published in 1952, four further editions followed: DSM II, DSM III, DSM III-R, and DSM IV. In each new edition, the list of psychiatric disorders continued to become longer and longer. The first edition defined 112 mental disorders, including brain disorders, psychotic disorders, neuroses of various sorts, personality disorders, and sexual deviation (including homosexuality). In 1968, the manual was revised and called DSM II. By now the number of disorders had jumped to 163.

"[I]f we were to follow logically the medical approach, almost everybody would be mentally 'ill.' The present official classification of psychiatric 'diseases' is already so broad that there is a real question whether anybody can claim to *not* fit into at least one category" (our italics), wrote psychiatrist E. Fuller Torrey in *The Death of Psychiatry* in 1974. "In short, all you have to do to qualify as 'normal' under the present system is to be a bowl of Jello."[4]

DSM II, however, was just the beginning. In fact, the real "growth" occurred in 1980 when the number of mental disorders reached the total of 224 in DSM III. Seven years later, in DSM III-R, it was increased to 253, while DSM IV, released in 1994, brought the number of mental diseases to the grand total of 374! Should this imply that society has, in three decades, become 300 percent more mentally ill? Or is Carol Tavris, author of *Mismeasure of Woman*, perhaps correct in stating that the authors of DSM suffer from "delusional scientific diagnosing disorder?"[5]

In DSM III, fourteen new sexual disorders were added, but noticeably homosexuality was removed from the manual as a form of deviancy. This change was not the result of any scientific discovery or advance. It was precipitated by active lobbying from the homosexual community. To decide the issue, the American Psychiatric Association took a vote from its membership. The result was 5,854 supporting and 3,810 opposed. On that basis, homosexuality went from a long-standing form of abnormal behavior to a scientifically-declared form of "sexual preference."[6]

In *Psychiatry: The Ultimate Betrayal*, the author Bruce Wiseman quotes psychiatrist Walter Afield: "I was just talking last weekend to somebody who was on the commission to do DSM IV that was coming out, and I said, 'Well now, tell me, homosexuality used to be considered a disease and then it was not considered a disease. What's it going to be in DSM IV?' And he said, 'Oh, we've totally cured it now. It doesn't exist.' "[7]

While homosexuality was voted "out," an increasing number of fabricated mental illnesses associated with children and adolescents, was voted "in." One psychologist, attending the DSM III-R hearings, described the intellectual effort put into the composition of the diagnostic manual as "shocking." "Diagnoses were developed by majority vote on the level we would choose a restaurant. You feel like Italian, I feel like Chinese, so let's go to a cafeteria. Then it's typed into the computer. It may reflect on our naivete, but it was our belief that there would be an attempt to look at things scientifically."[8]

In DSM II, a whole new category of "Behavior disorders of childhood and adolescence" made its appearance, listing seven disorders. In DSM III, thirty-two new disorders were added to this category. In DSM III, we also saw the birth of the now-notorious ADD.

Previously known under other names, ADD has grown from a relatively rare neurological condition to a mental illness, today said to afflict millions of children and adults. ADD (attention deficit disorder) or ADHD (attention deficit hyperactivity disorder), as it was renamed in DSM IV, has the support of thousands of so-called scientific studies, the American Psychiatric Association, the U.S. Department of Education, and many other institutions in the United States and worldwide. Yet, like Dr. Cartwright's "drapetomania," ADHD "may in fact come clothed in scientific respectability, yet have disturbing social overtones which are scarcely acknowledged by the wider educational community."[9]

A New Interpretation of An Old Problem

According to the medical view, ADHD is a syndrome characterized by a variety of symptoms, such as distractibility, a short attention span, poor concentration, daydreaming, restlessness, hyperactivity, and impulsiveness.

ADHD is a new interpretation of an old problem. The syndrome has changed names at least twenty-five times in the past 120 years.[10] During the 1930s and 1940s, up to about 1957, this syndrome was known as "hyperkinesis," a rare phenomenon with an incidence of perhaps one out of two thousand individuals. These rare individuals seemed to be driven by an inner whirlwind, not just in school, but constantly. They were always moving, climbing and knocking things over, and were in constant danger of injuring themselves or others.[11]

Unlike the hyperkinesis of the 1950s, and any other medical condition such as diabetes or pneumonia, ADHD pops up in one setting, only to disappear in another. The same child who has "ants in his pants" in the classroom, can be as quiet as a mouse in front of the television set. This reminds one of Cartwright's "drapetomania," which occurred in Negroes only *after* they had been captured.

Studies reveal that up to 80 percent of the time, children labeled ADHD do not appear to show symptoms of this disorder in several different real-life settings. First, up to 80 percent of them don't appear to be ADHD when in the physician's office. They also seem to behave normally in other unfamiliar settings where there is a one-to-one interaction with an adult. Second, they appear to be indistinguishable from so-called normals when they are in classrooms or other learning environments where children can choose their own learning activities and pace themselves through those experiences. Third, they seem to perform quite normally when they are paid to do specific activities designed to assess attention. Fourth, children labeled ADHD behave and attend quite normally when they are involved in activities that interest them and are novel in some way, or that involve high levels of stimulation. Finally, some of these children reach adulthood only to discover that the symptoms related to ADHD have apparently disappeared.[12]

If the incidences of symptoms related to ADHD are determined by situations, it is understandable that there are no laboratory tests, blood tests or brain scans to diagnose this disorder. Even the APA admits in its DSM IV that there are "no laboratory tests that have been established as diagnostic" for ADHD.[13] Nevertheless, one continually hears from or reads of parents, after seeking advice for their children's problems, that this or that test has "proven" their children to have ADHD. The truth is that this "abnormality" can only be inferred from comparing the child's behavior with vague and nonmedical measures, such as "is often forgetful in daily activities," or "often speaks excessively" (see table of criteria below).

According to the standards used in DSM III, before a child could be diagnosed as ADHD, at least six of the symptoms of inattention must have persisted for at least six months to a degree that is maladaptive and inconsistent with developmental level. In DSM IV, the authors of this manual have kindly created a category known as "ADHD Not Otherwise Specified." This category allows psychiatrists to diagnose ADHD more freely when a child's behavior doesn't fit the description. In other words, if a psychiatrist "senses" a child has the problem, he may say that he has it.[14]

With such vague criteria for ADHD, it is understandable, then, that prevalence figures for ADHD vary widely—far more widely than the 3 to 5 percent figure that popular books and articles use as a standard. In one epidemiological survey conducted in England, only two children out of 2,199 were diagnosed as hyperactive (.09 percent). Conversely, in Israel, 28 percent of children were rated by teachers as hyperactive. And in an earlier study in the United States, teachers rated 49.7 percent of boys as restless, 43.5 percent of boys as having a "short attention span," and 43.5 percent of boys as "inattentive to what others say."[15] "As with other psychiatric 'diseases,' the rate of diagnosis varies with the eagerness to diagnose it," says Vatz.[16] Evidently, if you only have a hammer in your hand, everything looks like a nail.

According to the *New England Journal of Medicine,* the diagnosis of ADHD and its treatment with medication may also be determined by cultural factors.[17] In a major report from the British Psychological Society, British physicians and psychologists were warned not to follow the Canadian and U.S. practice of applying the label ADHD to such a wide variety of behaviors in children. "The idea that children who don't attend or don't sit still in school have a mental disorder is not entertained by most British clinicians," the report stated.[18] This warning has clearly fallen on deaf ears. An armada of British psychiatrists and psychologists has recently begun to proclaim this "disease." The prescriptions for Ritalin in the United Kingdom have risen from two thousand in 1991 to ninety-two thousand in 1997. The National Health Service bill for Ritalin was £1,636,000 in 1997 and was expected to rise beyond £2,000,000 in 1998.[19]

DSM-IV Diagnostic Criteria for ADHD

Either 1 or 2:
1. Six or more of the following symptoms of inattention have persisted for at least six months to a degree that is maladaptive and inconsistent with developmental level:

a. Often fails to give close attention to details or makes careless mistakes in schoolwork, work, or other activities.
b. Often has difficulty sustaining attention in tasks or play activities.
c. Often does not seem to listen when spoken to directly.
d. Often does not follow through on instructions and fails to finish schoolwork, chores, or duties in the workplace (not due to oppositional behavior or failure to understand instructions).
e. Often has difficulty organizing tasks and activities.
f. Often avoids, dislikes, or is reluctant to engage in tasks that require sustained mental effort (such as homework).
g. Often loses things necessary for tasks or activities (toys, school assignments, pencils, books, or tools).
h. Is often easily distracted by extraneous stimuli.
i. Is often forgetful in daily activities.

2. Six or more of the following symptoms of hyperactivity-impulsivity have persisted for at least six months to a degree that is maladaptive and inconsistent with developmental level:

Hyperactivity:

a. Often fidgets with hands or feet or squirms in seat.
b. Often leaves seat in classroom or in other situations in which remaining seated is expected.
c. Often runs about or climbs excessively in situations in which it is inappropriate (in adolescents or adults, may be limited to subjective feelings of restlessness).
d. Often has difficulty playing or engaging in leisure activities quietly.
e. Is often "on the go" or often acts as if "driven by a motor."
f. Often talks excessively.

Impulsivity:

g. Often blurts out answers before questions have been completed.
h. Often has difficulty awaiting turn.
i. Often interrupts or intrudes on others (such as butting into conversations or games).

In Search of a Biological Cause

In order to substantiate the claim that ADHD is a disease, there must be a medical or biological cause for it. Yet, as with everything else about ADHD, none of its advocates is exactly sure what causes it. Possible biological causes that have been proposed include genetic factors, biochemical abnormalities (imbalances of such brain chemicals as serotonin, dopamine, and norepinephrine), neurological damage, lead poisoning, thyroid problems, prenatal exposure to various chemical agents, and delayed myelinization of the "nerve pathways of the brain."[20] Most parents are probably familiar with the term "biochemical imbalance in the brain," or "neurobiological disorder," the catchall phrases used in many consulting rooms to explain the cause of ADHD today.

A recently proposed cause that startled us is the suggestion that ADHD is the result of vaccinations. In fact, vaccines are not only proposed as being the cause of ADHD, but also of nearly every disease and of all social problems—whooping cough, polio-like paralysis, allergies, renal attacks, rheumatism, unexpected infant death, encephalitis, meningitis, Hepatitis B, autism, anorexia and bulimia, cerebral palsy, child leukemia, multiple sclerosis, cancer, AIDS, sterility, epilepsy, Parkinson's disease, cardiovascular illnesses, Alzheimer's, arthritis, late mental development, behavior problems, personality problems, learning problems, hypersexuality, emotional instability, juvenile delinquency, sociopathic personality, and criminal behavior. The list ends with the warning that vaccinations are a "threat of extinction for the human race."

There have been many medical substances in the past—and there still are—that were believed to be effective but were actually harmful. Thalidomide, for example, was introduced to the market in the 1950s to combat nausea and insomnia in pregnant women.

When taken in the first trimester of pregnancy, Thalidomide prevented the proper growth of the fetus, resulting in horrific birth defects in thousands of children around the world who were born during the late 1950s and early 1960s.[21]

Because of the Thalidomide tragedy (and many others), we found it hard to simply discard the allegations made by the anti-vaccinationists, as we thought there might be some vestige of truth in the idea. What amazed us though, was the distinct difference in statistics between the two sides—those for and against vaccinations. Take, for example, the DPT inoculation, which provides protection against diphtheria, pertussis (familiarly known as whooping cough) and tetanus. This shot, especially the vaccine against whooping cough, is viewed as the most dangerous of all the vaccinations. According to one anti-vaccination source, the incidence of whooping cough went up by 300 percent since DPT became mandatory in most American states in 1978. This source also stated that this vaccine "guarantees NO protection from the disease nor relief of its symptoms," and "those not vaccinated for it seem to have less severe symptoms than those who have been vaccinated."[22] A source of the pro-vaccine league, on the other hand, states that whooping cough killed five thousand to ten thousand people in the United States each year before a vaccine was available. Now the whooping cough vaccine has reduced the annual number of deaths to less than twenty per year.[23]

After a thorough investigation, we had to admit that there are some biological risks involved in vaccines. However, we decided that, should any of us have ten more children, we shall still have them all vaccinated. The chance of a tragedy is simply far smaller with vaccination than without it. In Japan, for example, after two children died from side effects in 1974 and 1975, the use of pertussis vaccine was banned for two months. Many parents were so alarmed that even after it was reinstated, they refused to inoculate their children. As a result, twenty-eight thousand Japanese children contracted whooping cough between 1977 and 1979, and ninety-three died. By comparison, between 1972 and 1974 Japan reported only 1,024 cases and six deaths.[24]

What we find ridiculous, however, is the suggestion that vaccines are responsible for all the world's social problems. Although we agree with the anti-vaccinationists that we are living in "a time in history unlike any before it, representing rebellion, immorality, drug and alcohol abuse, irresponsibility, disrespect for property and authority, impulsive behavior, crime, love of rebellious music, depression, anxiety, and violence towards others,"[25] vaccines are certainly not the cause. If so, Sweden would have solved at least some of their social problems by now, after banning pertussis vaccines in 1979. The contrary, however, is true. As in other Western countries, youth-related behavior and social problems in Sweden are steadily becoming more and more acute.

Like the vaccination scare, there are periodic "discoveries" that are advertised as the Rosetta stone for those seeking to define ADD or ADHD as a disease. The first "breakthrough" in treating hyperactive children came by a pediatrician and allergist, Dr. Benjamin Feingold. In *Why Your Child Is Hyperactive,* Dr. Feingold proposed that food additives, particularly synthetic flavors and colors in the diet, were related to hyperactivity and learning disabilities, as well as many other behavior problems in children. He reported that the elimination of all foods containing artificial colors and flavors, as well as salicylates and certain other additives, stopped the hyperactivity.

Dr. Feingold's book, which introduced his Feingold diet, received wide publicity. Because of the hope that he might be correct and a need to either counter his claims or to prove that he was correct, several research centers began to do research in this area. However, these hopes were soon dashed. According to Silver, the Feingold diet "is not effective in treating hyperactivity in most children. There may be a small percentage (1 to 2 percent) who appear to respond positively to the diet for reasons that are not yet clear. There is no way for the physician to identify in advance which patients might be part of this small percentage."[26]

In its search for a physical cause, the ADHD movement reached another milestone with the publication in the *New England Journal of Medicine* of a study by Alan Zametkin and his colleagues at the National Institute of Mental Health. This study appeared to link hyperactivity in adults with reduced metabolism of glucose (a prime energy source) in the premotor cortex and the superior prefrontal cortex—areas of the brain involved in the control of attention, planning, and motor activity. In other words, these areas of the brain were not working as hard as they should have been, according to Zametkin.[27] Armstrong continues:

> The media picked up on Zametkin's research and reported it nationally. ADD proponents latched on to this study as "proof" of the medical basis for ADD. Pictures depicting the spread of glucose through a "normal" brain compared to a "hyperactive" brain began showing up in CH.A.D.D. (Children and Adults with Attention Deficit Disorder) literature and at the organization's conventions and meetings. One ADD advocate seemed to speak for many in the ADD movement when she wrote: "In November 1990, parents of children with ADD heaved a collective sigh of relief when Dr. Alan Zametkin released a report that hyperactivity (which is closely linked to ADD) results from an insufficient rate of glucose metabolism in the brain. Finally, commented a supporter, we have an answer to skeptics who pass this off as bratty behavior caused by poor parenting."
>
> What was not reported by the media or cheered by the ADD community was the study by Zametkin and others

that came out three years later in the *Archives of General Psychiatry*. In an attempt to repeat the 1990 study with adolescents, the researchers found no significant differences between the brains of so-called hyperactive subjects and those of so-called normal subjects. And in retrospect, the results of the first study didn't look good either. When the original 1990 study was controlled for sex (there were more men in the hyperactive group than in the control group), there was no significant difference between groups.[28]

A recent critique of Zametkin's research by faculty members of the University of Nebraska also pointed out that the study did not make clear whether the lower glucose rates found in "hyperactive brains" were a cause or a result of attention problems. The critics pointed out that if subjects were startled and then had their levels of adrenaline monitored, adrenaline levels would probably be quite high. We would not say, however, that these individuals had an adrenaline disorder. Rather, we'd look at the underlying conditions that led to abnormal adrenaline levels. Similarly, even if biochemical differences did exist in the so-called hyperactive brain, we ought to be looking at the non-biological factors that could account for some of these differences, including stress, learning style, and temperament.[29]

Despite the complete lack of proof that ADHD has a medical cause (just as "drapetomania" was never proven to be a disease), the disorder has burgeoned—considering only the United States—from 500 thousand diagnoses in 1988 to 4.4 million in 1997.[30] The inability of researchers to prove that ADHD has a biological cause actually confirms, time and time again, that other factors, such as the environment or education, are playing a role.

"The past twenty-five years has led to a phenomenon almost unique in history," says McGuinness. "Methodological rigorous research . . . indicates that ADD (attention deficit disorder) and hyperactivity as 'syndromes' simply do not exist. We [referring to psychiatry] have invented a disease, given it medical sanction, and now must disown it. The major question is how we go about destroying the monster we have created. It is not easy to do this and still save face.[31]

Based on a Logical Flaw

Problems with learning and behavior in children are certainly not a new phenomenon. Long before ADHD was inserted in the

DSM, teachers and parents had been complaining that some children are difficult to teach and control, that they underachieve academically or can't sit still. Even as early as 400 B.C. Socrates complained about teenagers who "love luxury, have bad manners, have contempt for authority, disrespect their elders, and love to chatter in places of exercise."[32] Problems with children are thus not new, but the fashion to attribute common problems to biochemical or neurological abnormalities and to describe these affected children as victims of a medical syndrome or mental disorder, certainly is.[33]

Despite the inability of researchers to find any proof for their claim that ADHD is a disease, this theory has, through repeating it over and over, taken on the authority of proven fact. In fact, it is probably more accurate to call this idea a myth than a theory. The difference between the two is that the former is a *fabricated story*, whereas the latter is an attempt to give a *scientific explanation* for a phenomenon. The ancient Greeks, for example, could not find a rational explanation for the daily movement of the sun through the heavens. They fabricated the story of Helios and his fiery chariot. The Egyptians, on the other hand, who were likewise unable to find a rational explanation for the movement of the sun, pictured their sun god Ra as a scarab pushing the sun across the sky. Today, thanks to the work of scientists like Galileo, Kepler, and Copernicus, every schoolchild knows that the sun only *appears* to be moving through the skies. It is actually the movement of the earth that creates this illusion.

To have a better understanding of how this ridiculous idea—that a behavior problem can be blamed on a biological deficit—has become a "scientific fact," it is necessary to go back in history to the time when these ideas originated. The present can only be fully understood if one examines its roots in the past. In this case, the key to comprehension resides in the research done by two German refugees, the psychiatrist Alfred Strauss and the psychologist Heinz Werner. These two scholars were employed during the late 1930s at the Wayne County Training School in Northville, Michigan, a school for educable mentally retarded (EMR) children.

While Strauss and Werner were employed at the school, they came to believe that their EMR students were of two basic types. The first group was the "endogenous type" and consisted of children who had a family history of mental deficiency. The "exogenous type," on the other hand, had no family history of mental deficiency, and according to Strauss and Werner their retardation was caused by brain injury—before, during or after birth. In comparing endogenous and exogenous children on perceptual and cognitive tasks, they found the endogenous group to be more successful than the brain-injured children regarding these abilities. The endogenous children had no behavioral problems, while the brain-injured children engaged in—what they described as—disturbed, unrestrained and volatile behavior. Also, endogenous children exhibited a small increase in their IQ scores during their stay at the Wayne County Training School, while exogenous children displayed a small decrease. They concluded that the IQ changes indicated that the curriculum for the mentally retarded was ineffective for the brain-damaged children.[34]

A few years later, Strauss and another coworker, Newell Kephart, expanded the study of brain injury to include children of normal intelligence. They argued that the kind of perceptual-motor, cognitive, and behavior problems that Strauss and Werner had found among the exogenous group were not only to be found in mentally defective children. These problems were also found in children of normal intelligence. On these grounds, they concluded that children of normal intelligence who exhibited these kinds of learning and behavior problems were brain damaged.[35]

Any person with even a basic knowledge of logic will know that a conclusion such as that of Strauss and Kephart is a logical flaw. The statement "people who do not have feet do not wear shoes," which is true, cannot simply be reversed into "people who do not wear shoes do not have feet." That, however, is exactly what Strauss and Kephart did. They simply reversed the statement "brain-damaged individuals exhibit learning and behavior problems," which is true, to "individuals who exhibit learning and behavior problems are brain damaged." Goodman used another analogy to point out this logical flaw: a drought can kill vegetation. If, however, we find dead vegetation, we cannot assume that drought was the cause. The vegetation could have been destroyed not by drought but by any number of causes including non-biological ones such as lumbering.[36] If a brain-damaged person exhibits certain characteristics, we cannot simply jump to the conclusion that a person is brain damaged when we see him exhibiting the same characteristics. There may be many other reasons for his behavior.

The research of Strauss and Werner has been criticized by many. Kenneth Kavale of the University of Iowa and Steven Forness of the University of California, for example, reanalyzed Strauss and Werner's original studies on brain-injured children. They concluded that the performance differences reported between the two groups of children—the "endogenous" and "exogenous"—were in fact too small to justify the distinction which Strauss and Werner had made.[37]

There was, furthermore, a critical problem involved in their research. Neither Strauss and Werner in their initial research with mentally defective children, nor Strauss and Kephart in their studies of children with normal intelligence, provided evidence of brain damage or other neurological dysfunctions. The brain damage was inferred *only* from the children's behavior.[38]

The Restoration of Status and Riddance of Guilt Feelings

The work of Strauss and Kephart has been continued by others. They also could prove neither brain damage nor neurological abnormalities in otherwise "normal" children, but the idea became more and more popular. In time, however, the term "brain damage" was changed to a less harmful syndrome called "minimal brain dysfunction." A few years later, this term also fell into disfavor in educational circles, and in 1963 the term "learning disabilities" (LD) was adopted. By 1980, the term ADD was established to refer to the "learning disability" that afflicts children who cannot pay attention, fidget, and do not listen when spoken to.

In spite of the inability of experts to prove any neurological dysfunction, middle-class parents, especially, accepted this diagnosis with great relief. Before the 1960s, learning problems in school were routinely attributed to emotional problems caused by the parents. Children were frequently misdiagnosed as mentally retarded and had to live with this stigma for the rest of their lives. One cannot but sympathize with the parents and the children of that time. "You felt like you were all alone," one parent said, "and no one could help. The educators made you feel like your child was a freak, and most of the medical people just didn't understand."[39]

Many middle-class parents thought that special education classifications such as "mentally retarded" and "emotionally disturbed" and prevailing social science categories for explaining academic failure such as "culturally deprived" seemed appropriate for children from minority and poor communities, but not for children from the middle class:

> The variety of problems afflicting minority groups and the poor were said to affect the emotions and intellect of children in ways that explained their difficulties in school. An

applicable but *different* explanation was needed for children who had grown up in the suburbs, with the advantages of middle-class life, and who, despite their academic problems, often appeared to be good learners outside of school. The learning disabilities explanation—that the problem was caused not by retardation or other exclusionary factors, but by a minor neurological "glitch"—made sense to many. The explanation also offered different advantages to different interests: it was less pejorative than other special-education categories and it did not consider or criticize any role schools, families, or other social influences might have had in creating the learning disabilities.[40]

Unfortunately, this new idea caused middle-class parents not only to rid themselves of guilt feelings, but also of their responsibilities toward their children. Within a few years after ideas of minimal brain dysfunction and learning disability had taken root, it became not only the cause of poor school achievement, but of nearly any physical or psychological problem, and simply any form of behavior that adults found troublesome, including children who were physically immature or advanced for their age, juvenile delinquents, children who would not listen to adults, who cried, hated, were aggressive, stuttered, had poor eating habits, had nightmares, wet their beds, bit their nails, sucked their thumbs, ran away from home, didn't keep their rooms neat, wouldn't take baths or brush their teeth, or teased the family cat. A dysfunction inside the brain became the scapegoat even for the parents' problems. Nancy Ramos, once president of the California Association for Neurologically Handicapped Children, echoes the message: "A good many LD children come from single-parent homes, but it's not the broken marriages that cause LD, it's that the learning-disabled child broke up the marriage in the first place."[41]

Notes

1. Armstrong, T., "ADD as a social invention," *Education Week,* 18 October 1995.

2. Ibid.

3. Syverud, M., "Don't stop the insanity (my therapist needs the money)," *Daily Messenger,* 13 August 1995, cited in B. Wiseman, *Psychiatry: The Ultimate Betrayal* (Los Angeles: Freedom Publishing, 1995), 357-358.

4. Torrey, E. F., *The Death of Psychiatry* (Radnor, PA: Little, Brown and Company, 1974), 54.

5. Baughman, F., Jr., "The future of mental health: Radical changes ahead," *USA Today*, vol. 125, 1 March 1997, 60.

6. Caplan, P. J., *They Say You're Crazy* (New York: Addison-Wesley Publishing Company, 1995), 165-167, cited in Wiseman, *Psychiatry: The Ultimate Betrayal*, 352.

7. Wiseman, *Psychiatry: The Ultimate Betrayal*, 352.

8. Caplan, *They Say You're Crazy*, 222, cited in Wiseman, *Psychiatry: The Ultimate Betrayal*, 354.

9. Armstrong, "ADD as a social invention."

10. Armstrong, T., "ADD: Does it really exist?" *Phi Delta Kappan*, February 1996.

11. Schrag, P., & Divoky, D., *The Myth of the Hyperactive Child and Other Means of Child Control* (Middlesex: Penguin Books, 1975).

12. Armstrong, "ADD: Does it really exist?"

13. *Diagnostic and Statistical Manual of Mental Disorders* (DSM IV), (Washington, DC: American Psychiatric Association, 1994).

14. Vatz, R. E., "Attention Deficit Delirium," *Wall Street Journal*, 27 July 1994.

15. Armstrong, "ADD: Does it really exist?"

16. Vatz, "Attention Deficit Delirium."

17. Ibid.

18. McConnell, H., "ADHD just doesn't add up to Brit psych society," *The Medical Post*, 21 January 1997.

19. Woolf, M., " 'Zombie drug' doses soaring," *Independent on Sunday*, 29 November 1998.

20. Armstrong, "ADD: Does it really exist?"

21. Talen, J., "Thalidomide's legacy; As new uses emerge for this infamous drug, people damaged by it are offering powerful reminders of its potential harm," *The Washington Post*, 4 January 2000.

22. Thompson, D., "Do vaccinations cause learning disabilities and behavioral problems?" 1997, website.

23. www.kidshealth.org, website.

24. Murphy, J. "Medicine: A comeback for whooping cough. Fear of vaccine mounts, and the number of cases doubles," *Time,* 30 June 1986.

25. Thompson, "Do vaccinations cause learning disabilities and behavioral problems?"

26. Silver, L. B., "The 'magic cure': A review of the current controversial approaches for treating learning disabilities," *Journal of Learning Disabilities,* vol. 20(8), 1987, 498-504.

27. Armstrong, "ADD: Does it really exist?"

28. Ibid.

29. Ibid.

30. Baughman, "The future of mental health."

31. McGuinness, D., "Attention deficit disorder: The emperor's new clothes, animal 'pharm,' and other fiction," in S. Fisher & R. P. Greenberg (eds.), *The Limits of Biological Treatments for Psychological Distress* (Hillsdale, NJ: Lawrence Erlbaum Associates, 1989), 151-188.

32. Malbon, A., "Dealing with teenage dramas," *Progress Press,* 19 October 1998, 8.

33. Schrag & Divoky, *The Myth of the Hyperactive Child.*

34. Franklin, B. M., "From brain injury to learning disability: Alfred Strauss, Heinz Werner and the historical development of the learning disabilities field," in B. M. Franklin (ed.), *Learning Disability: Dissenting Essays* (Philadelphia: The Farmer Press, 1987), 9-46.

35. Ibid.

36. Goodman, J. F., "Organicity as a construct in psychological diagnosis," in T. R. Kratochwill (ed.), *Advances in School Psychology,* vol. 3, (Hillsdale: Lawrence Erlbaum, 1983), 101-139.

37. Kavale, K. A., & Forness, S. R., "The historical foundation of learning disabilities: A quantitative synthesis assessing the validity of Strauss and Werner's exogenous versus endogenous distinction of mental retardation," *Remedial and Special Education,* vol. 65, 1985, 18-25; Kavale, K. A., & Forness, S. R., *The Science of Learning Disabilities* (San Diego, CA: College Hill Press, 1985), 54-60.

38. Franklin, "From brain injury to learning disability."

39. Schrag & Divoky, *The Myth of the Hyperactive Child.*

40. Coles, G., *The Learning Mystique* (New York: Pantheon Books, 1987), xiii.

41. Schrag & Divoky, *The Myth of the Hyperactive Child.*

3.

The "Smart Pill"

One afternoon last May, hundreds of schoolchildren in Peoria, Illinois, rallied against drug abuse at a park just outside of the city. Wearing scarlet "Dare To Say No To Drugs" T-shirts, they celebrated Drug Abuse Resistance Education day—DARE day—with volleyball, tug of war, and soda pop. Cars in the parking lot, watched over by cops on horseback, were plastered with DARE bumper stickers. In the schools during the year, each class had its own DARE police officer who regularly volunteered to teach lessons on the horrors of drugs. Yet, in this most conservative of Midwestern cities, somewhere between 5 percent and 8 percent of the schoolchildren take, with the school district's blessing, a powerful stimulant to help them get through each day.[1]

This "powerful stimulant" in question is Ritalin (methylphenidate). Nicknamed "kiddie cocaine" by psychologist John Breeding, Ritalin is widely prescribed to overactive kids. Even school officials endorse the drug, making it hard for worried parents to "just say no."

The production of Ritalin increased sixfold in the U.S. from 1990 to 1996. According to a report issued by the U.N.'s Vienna-based International Narcotics in February 1996, as many as 5 percent of all American schoolchildren—and 12 percent of all boys between the ages of six and fourteen—are being treated with Ritalin.[2]

The school of the 1990s in Queensland, Australia, is one where children no longer line up for milk, but queue for drugs to control their behavior problems. It is not a job enjoyed by all. As one teacher remarked, "As an early childhood teacher, it breaks my heart to have to administer [these drugs] to children as young as three and then to see them spend their day in a zombie-like state."[3] In Australia, the prescription rate of Dexedrine, a stimulant in the same class as Ritalin, soared from 9,937 in 1990 to 127,377 in 1995.[4] Ritalin prescriptions jumped from 23,340 in 1990 to 295,700 in 1997.[5]

In America—and elsewhere—Ritalin is considered a controlled substance, a fact not widely known. A drug becomes a controlled substance when it has the potential for abuse and/or addiction. Other drugs in the same category are cocaine, opium, and morphine. Due to the excessive dosage of children with a controlled substance, the controversy surrounding Ritalin has been going on for a long time.

On 29 September 1970, the Committee on Government Operations of the U.S. House of Representatives voiced their concern that two hundred thousand to three hundred thousand children were already being drugged, and the committee correctly surmised that eventually the figures would soar. The committee noted the irony that "each and every school child is told that 'speed kills,' " while many children are being forced to take speed in the form of Ritalin. It warned about the effect of this on "our extensive national campaign against drug abuse." Testimony was received about a pattern of teachers and school administrators intimidating parents into giving Ritalin to their children.[6]

As the drug makes many kids who have been bouncing off walls and talking incessantly sit still, listen, and focus, the intimidation from harassed teachers trying to cope with large and undisciplined classes is—quite understandably—continuing. It is not uncommon in many U.S. classrooms today to find 20 percent of the children on Ritalin, and the numbers are multiplying. The drug has become such a common element of schooling that the *New Yorker* magazine listed it as one of the three R's—"Readin, Ritin, Ritalin"—on its cover.

One of the concerns in the use of stimulants is that they often have side effects, the most commonly reported being the loss of appetite, serious weight loss, insomnia, depression, headaches, stomachaches, bed-wetting, irritability, and dizziness. Reports also indicate severe psychological effects. A large percentage of children become robotic, lethargic, depressed, or withdrawn on stimulants, and withdrawal from them can cause emotional suffering, including depression, exhaustion, and suicide.[7] According to the DSM III-R, published in 1987, "suicide is the major complication" of withdrawal from Ritalin and similar drugs.

In 1995, Denmark's Cooperative Institute for Medical Drug Dependence reported the following withdrawal symptoms from psychotropic drug dependence: "Emotional changes: fear, terror, panic, fear of insanity, failing self-confidence, restlessness, irritability, aggression, an urge to destroy, and, in the worst cases, an urge to kill."[8]

Psychotic episodes and violent behavior are also associated with chronic Ritalin abuse. Even the manufacturer warns in its information leaflet, "frank psychotic episodes may occur" with abuse.

The history of violence by teens who have been subjected to psychiatric drugs cannot be ignored. One example is that of Kip Kinkel, who went on a wild shooting spree at his Springfield, Oregon high school on 21 May 1998 that left two dead and twenty-two injured. Kip also shot his parents, killing them. Was it merely Kip's anger—he had been attending anger control classes—that got the better of him? Or were the Prozac and Ritalin he was reportedly taking at least partially responsible? Could this incident have been prevented?

In his book *Talking Back to Ritalin,* psychiatrist Dr. Peter R. Breggin documents other side effects, which he claims have been confirmed by scientific studies but are ignored by the advocates of Ritalin. He states that Ritalin can retard growth in children by disrupting the cycles of growth hormone released by the pituitary gland. According to Breggin, the drug routinely causes gross malfunctions in the brain of the child. There is research evidence from a few controlled studies that Ritalin can cause shrinkage (atrophy) or other permanent physical abnormalities in the brain.[9]

Perhaps the most controversial issue in the Ritalin debate is the question whether its use can lead to psychological drug dependence in the long run. A study in the *Archives of General Psychiatry* titled "Is methylphenidate like cocaine?" concluded that indeed it was. Its lead author, Nora Volkow, director of nuclear medicine at the Brookhaven National Laboratory in Upton, N.Y., used positron emission tomography scans to look at where and how quickly Ritalin acts in the brain. In Volkow's study, eight healthy male volunteers were injected with the drug. Their scans were then compared with those subjects in previous studies who had been injected with cocaine. The authors reported that the distribution of Ritalin in the human brain was "almost identical to that of cocaine." The drugs' effects also peaked at almost the same time—between four and ten minutes in the case of Ritalin, and two to eight minutes for cocaine. Even the highs were similar.

When Ritalin was given to cocaine users, they said it was "almost indistinguishable." The only significant difference was that Ritalin took more than four times as long—ninety minutes—to leave the body. "We're dealing with a drug that does have properties very similar to cocaine," Volkow concluded.[10]

It is therefore quite understandable why Ritalin—nicknamed "Vitamin R," "The R Ball," or "The Smart Pill"—has become the drug of choice in American middle schools, where kids share their own prescriptions or sell pills to friends who crush them up and snort the powder for a quick high. The result has been increased drug dealing among the young, plus several teen deaths. In 1991, fewer than twenty-five children, aged ten to fourteen, were admitted to emergency rooms for methylphenidate abuse. In 1995, the number climbed above four hundred—about the same as for cocaine abusers in that age group.[11] Worse, young children on the drug may be terrorized by teens looking for a hit.

Although taking a stimulant orally is very different from injecting or snorting it, there are warnings that, even when taken orally, its use has the potential of creating long-term drug dependence. According to psychopharmacologist Susan Schenk of Texas A&M University, children treated with Ritalin are three times more likely to develop a taste for cocaine. She reached this conclusion after teaming up with Nadine Lambert, a developmental psychologist at the University of California, Berkeley, who followed children with ADHD from adolescence to adulthood.[12]

"The early exposure to a stimulant makes the brain more receptive to other drugs," says Dr. Denis Donovan, a child psychiatrist.[13] "Ritalin is becoming the 'gateway drug' that leads kids into later drug use," adds psychologist John Breeding.[14]

Discouraging Results

If stimulant treatment achieved positive results, one could surely ignore its critics and even rationalize its side effects. That, however, does not seem to be the case. In a study entitled "Hyperactive Children as Teenagers: A Follow-up Study" (1971), eighty-three children were followed from two to five years after being diagnosed as hyperactive or as having attention deficit disorder. Ninety-two percent of the children were treated with Ritalin. Results were as follows:

- 60% of the children were still overactive and had poor schoolwork (the original reasons for being put on Ritalin), but in addition were now viewed as rebellious;

- 59% had had some contact with the police;

- 23% had been taken to the police station one or more times;

- 58% had failed one or more grades;

- 57% had reading difficulties;

- 44% had arithmetic difficulties;

- 78% found it hard to sit still and study;

- 59% were viewed as a discipline problem at school;

- 83% had trouble with frequent lying;

- 52% were destructive;

- 34% had threatened to kill their parents;

- 15% had talked of or attempted suicide.[15]

Another research study, the Satterfield study (1987), states,

> We found juvenile delinquency rates to be 20-25 times greater in our hyperactive drug-treated only group than in the normal control group. In the "Delinquency outcome for the drug-treated group," the results were: of 61 boys, 46% were arrested for one or more felony offenses before age 18; 30% were arrested for two or more felony offenses; 25% were institutionalized. . . . Studies of the long-term effectiveness of drugs have been consistently discouraging.[16]

There is also scant evidence of improved academic performance with stimulant treatment. According to Rooney, research has still not shown the use of medication to be significantly effective in the treatment of processing deficits or academic achievement.[17] In *The Learning Mystique,* Professor Gerald Coles confirms the findings of a 1978 review of both short- and long-term studies on the use of stimulants with children who were hyperactive and learning disabled. Of a total of seventeen studies included in this review, short- or long-term, whether they met basic scientific criteria or not, all the conclusions agreed: "stimulant drugs have little, if any, impact on . . . long-term academic improvement." Their major effect seemed to be an "improvement in classroom manageability."[18]

In the *Journal of Behavioral Optometry* (1991), a study evaluated twenty-two previous studies/articles since 1976 concerning Ritalin use for hyperactive children. It states:

> The fact that the above studies do not show the efficacy of Ritalin for helping hyperactive children should be apparent to the skeptic and make a skeptic out of the believer. But the argument should not stop at this point. The weak evidence for the value of Ritalin must now be viewed in the light of its reported side effects.

According to Dr. Fred A. Baughman, Jr., a children's neurologist, Ritalin's lack of effectiveness has been proved by hundreds of studies but has not been revealed to doctors, teachers, or parents. Instead, its manufacturer spends millions of dollars to sell parent groups and doctors on the idea of using Ritalin. C.H.A.D.D., with six hundred chapters and 35,000 members in America, has received nearly one million dollars from Ritalin's manufacturer, a Swiss-owned company formerly known as Ciba-Geigy and recently renamed Novartis. In return, C.H.A.D.D.'s message to the public unfailingly portrays that ADHD is a real disease "like a brain tumor or diabetes," and Ritalin is "safe and non-addictive."[19]

Our subjective experience is that stimulant treatment is indeed successful in improving a number of children's behaviors and academic performance in the short term. This number, however, is minuscule and its use hard to justify if one considers its possible side effects and the results obtained in the long term. For most children, "successful treatment" seems to imply maintenance, by providing a robotic or zombie-like state. Mark Stewart, a child psychiatrist at the University of Iowa, remarked in an interview:

> They come off the drugs at fourteen or so, and suddenly they're big, strong people who've never had to spend any time building any controls in learning how to cope with their own daily stress. Then the parents, who have forgotten what the child's real personality was like without the mask of the drug, panic and say: "Help me, I don't know what to do with him. He's taller than I am and he has the self-discipline of a six-year-old." At that point the parent sees the only solution as going back to the drug. They can only deal with the medicated child. That's the seductiveness of successful drug treatment—that it temporarily solves the problem without asking the people involved to do anything.[20]

"Parents and teachers and even doctors have been badly misled by drug company marketing practices," says psychiatrist Peter Breggin. "Drug companies have targeted children as a big market likely to boost profits—and children are suffering as a result."

"Our society has institutionalized drug abuse among our children," Breggin adds:

> Worse yet, we abuse our children with drugs rather than making an effort to find better ways to meet their needs. In the long run, we are giving our children a very bad lesson— that drugs are the answer to emotional problems. We are encouraging a generation of youngsters to grow up relying on psychiatric drugs rather than on themselves and other human resources. . . . attention deficit disorder does not reflect children's deficits but our lack of attention to their needs.[21]

Notes

1. Ruenzel, B., "ADDicted," *Editorial Projects in Education,* November/ December 1996.

2. Barber, S., "High on discipline," *Sunday Times,* 3 March 1996.

3. "The sacred cows of psychiatric drugs: Child drug pushing," *Psychiatry: Betraying and Drugging Children* (Los Angeles: CCHR, 1998), 12- 15.

4. Ibid.

5. Figures from Commonwealth Department of Health and Family Services, Australia.

6. Breggin, P. R., *Toxic Psychiatry: Why Therapy, Empathy and Love Must Replace the Drugs, Electroshock, and Biochemical Theories of the New Psychology* (Martin's Press: New York, 1991).

7. Breggin, P. R., *Talking Back to Ritalin. What Doctors Aren't Telling You about Stimulants for Children* (Common Courage Press, 1998).

8. "Ruthless kids: Psychiatric drugs cause violence," *Psychiatry: Betraying and Drugging Children* (Los Angeles: CCHR, 1998), 16-17.

9. Breggin, *Talking Back to Ritalin.*

10. Motluk, A., "Health Institute conference will study Ritalin's kinship

to cocaine," *Minneapolis Star Tribune,* 30 April 1998.

11. Lang, J., "Ritalin nation: Little boys on drugs," *Scripps Howard News Service,* www.dailyparent.com/dailyp/source/article/1638.html.

12. Motluk, "Health Institute conference will study Ritalin's kinship to cocaine."

13. Lang, "Ritalin nation."

14. Russell, J., "The pill that teachers push," *Good Housekeeping,* vol. 225, 1 December 1997.

15. Mendelson, W., Johnson, N., and Stewart, M. A., "Hyperactive children as teenagers: A follow-up study," *Journal of Nervous Mental Disorders,* vol. 153, 1971.

16. Satterfield, J. H., Satterfield, B. T., and Schnell, A. M., "Therapeutic interventions to prevent delinquency in hyperactive boys," *Journal of the American Academy of Child and Adolescence Psychiatry,* vol. 26(1), 1987, 56-64.

17. Rooney, K. J., "Controversial therapies: A review and critique," *Intervention in School and Clinic,* vol. 26(3), 1991, 134-142.

18. Barkley, R. A., & Cunningham, C. E., "Do stimulant drugs improve the academic performance of hyperkinetic children?" *Clinical Pediatrics,* vol. 17, 1978: 85-92, cited in Coles, G., *The Learning Mystique* (New York: Pantheon Books, 1987), 94.

19. Baughman, F., Jr., "The future of mental health: Radical changes ahead," *USA Today,* vol. 125, 1 March 1997, 60.

20. Schrag, P., & Divoky, D., *The Myth of the Hyperactive Child and Other Means of Child Control* (Middlesex: Penguin Books, 1975).

21. Breggin, P. R., www.breggin.com.

4.

Man Must Learn to Be Human

When he was found in a forest in the late eighteenth century, he was completely naked, gathering acorns and roots to eat. Eventually the boy was captured and brought back to civilization. The boy was given the name Victor and is often referred to as the Wild Boy of Aveyron.

Victor's tutor, Itard, describes the behavior of the boy and his own efforts to teach him to do the things ordinary human beings do, including speaking and reading. The boy was eleven or twelve years of age when he was found, and could not speak at all. He grunted and trotted like an animal and scratched those who opposed him. Victor's tutor tells us that his senses were extraordinarily apathetic. His nostrils were filled with snuff without making him sneeze. He picked up potatoes from boiling water. A pistol fired near him provoked hardly any response, though the sounds of cracking a walnut caused him to turn around.

Itard tried to teach Victor to speak and read. At the end of five years, Victor could identify some written words and phrases referring to objects and actions, and even some words referring to simple relationships such as big and small, and he could use word cards to indicate some of his desires. However, he did not learn to speak.

There were many people at that time who regarded Victor simply as having been born mentally defective and therefore incapable of acquiring more language than he did. However, it would be difficult to explain how a mentally defective child could have been able to fend for himself in the wilds for any length of time. The question should rather be asked: what *method* did Itard use to teach Victor?

A more recent story of children growing up in isolation from other humans is that of Amala and Kamala. In 1920, as the story goes, the Rev. Singh saw a mother wolf and cubs, two of whom had long, matted hair and looked human. After considerable preparations and difficulties, the two human creatures were captured. They turned out to be two girls whose ages were assessed by Singh at about eight years and one and a half years.

Singh described them as "wolfish" in appearance and behavior. They walked on all fours and had calluses on their knees and palms from doing so. They prowled and howled at night. For a long time they remained fond of raw meat and stole it when the occasion offered. They slept rolled up in a bundle on the floor, they resisted the approaches of human beings, and they did not speak. Their tongues permanently hung out of their thick, red lips, and they panted just like wolves. They licked all liquids with their tongues, and ate their food in a crouched position. With regard to the development of their senses, it was noted that their hearing was very acute and that they could smell meat at a great distance. Furthermore, they could orient themselves very well at night. Amala, the younger, died within a year, but Kamala lived until 1929.

By means of intimate and devoted contact with Kamala, by softening her skin with oil and massaging her, by feeding and caressing her, Mrs. Singh was able to win her confidence and to create the conditions in which Kamala would be willing to learn from her. For a long time Kamala preferred the company of cats and dogs to that of children. In the end, she came to enjoy children more and more, but never became easy and secure.

She needed considerable training to stand erect, and could only do so for the first time twenty months after having been found. By January 1926, she had learned to walk erect, and for the remaining two years of her life, though her movements remained somewhat wolflike, she showed quite clearly that her previous way of walking had been due merely to the absence of ordinary human training.

As far as language development is concerned, her first recorded attempt at imitating a word spoken by people around her came two years and two months after she had been rescued. After six years of living with human beings, she had a vocabulary of thirty-six to forty words, and from then on she learned quite a few words and phrases, and even started to speak in sentences. However, until her death, her language remained very rudimentary and was confined to concrete and immediate situations.[1]

Other stories of children raised by animals include a boy who was found in Mozambique, an African state, in 1968. When found, a female baboon tried to protect him. It was believed that he had been living among the baboons for eighteen years. He had even learned to swing from tree to tree. There is also the story of a boy who lived in Syria, who ate grass and could leap like an antelope, as well as of a girl, who lived in the forests of Indonesia for six years after she had fallen into the river. She walked like an ape and her teeth were as sharp as razors.[2]

If one reads these stories, one simply has to agree with Ashley Montagu that being human is not a status *with* which, but *to* which, one is born. While every creature that is classified physically as man is thereby called *Homo sapiens*, no such creature is really *human* until he or she exhibits the behavior characteristics of a human being. He, however, adds that one cannot deny the status of being human to a newborn baby because it cannot talk, cannot walk erect or reveal any of the other behavior characteristics of human beings. The way in which he reconciles this apparent contradiction with his previous statement is by pointing to the *promise* the child shows of being able to develop the behavior characteristics of human beings. The wonderful thing about a baby is its promise, not its performance—a promise that can only come true with the required help and assistance. The development of *Homo sapiens*, however great the promise might be, into a human being with behavior characteristics of human beings, requires more than just being kept alive physically. A child only becomes a human being thanks to *education*.[3]

Education starts at birth and continues as an interactional relationship between a more mature person (especially the mother and father, but also other adults such as teachers) who cares for the child and cannot escape his role as educator, and a less mature person (infant, child, young person) who attaches himself to the more mature person and inevitably is the one being educated. The educational relationship is a very special form of human relationship. We have no choice about educating and being educated, though of course we may educate badly and be badly educated.[4]

The term *education* requires some comment. Most people have come to identify education only with schools and schooling. The school has grown from the modest institution it was in the nineteenth century to one that is blamed for all the ills of society and is seen as potentially capable of curing them. The school's functions and influence have been extended (some would say overextended) and therefore the school is exceedingly vulnerable to criticism.[5] It is, however, very important to note that the whole of education does not take place in the school. It is especially responsible for the formal aspects of education, namely subject instruction, in order to provide society with an able workforce. The parents, on the other hand, are the *primary* educators of their children.

Apparently, the problem with children is that they come without operating instructions. It doesn't seem as if there is an accompanying manual, explaining to mothers how to handle toddlers who throw temper tantrums in the middle of busy shopping centers, or how fathers should react when their instructions are ignored or refused. Without the right instructions for situations like these, parenthood can become one long rollercoaster ride.

In the past, the knowledge and experience needed to raise and educate children were passed on among families and communities and down through the generations so that a recognizable tradition of child rearing can be seen almost anywhere one cares to look throughout history. These traditions were aimed at teaching a child to be unselfish rather than selfish; of expressing kind emotions instead of just feeling them; and of being able to control one's actions sufficiently to live up to one's ideas of good behavior and to accommodate the ways of others.[6] The last few decades, however, have seen an interruption of these traditions, says Burrows in her book, *Good Children*:

> Instead of the task of handing on skills being left to the men and women who have done the job themselves, and often on a grand scale, a new breed of experts has been encouraged to come to the fore. Many of these people, though often qualified in medicine and psychology, have never actually reared a family. And haven't they managed to make the whole thing seem difficult![7]

Hand in hand, psychology and its medical equal, psychiatry, have succeeded in replacing these time-honored traditions of childcare with—as Burrows calls them—ideas that are "ridiculous and outlandish." These ideas, sold to parents as "child-centered" educational styles, have confused parents and stripped them of their ability to take the lead in their own homes and produce healthy and secure children.

The Bandwagon that Went to a Funeral

Behaviorist J. B. Watson was one of the first of the "new breed of experts" that appeared on the scene. He offered what he called a "foolproof" method of child rearing, and mothers bought it hook, line, and sinker. If only they would follow his advice, he said, they could produce any kind of child they wanted—"a doctor, lawyer, artist, merchant-chief, and—yes—even a beggarman and a thief."[8]

In his book, *Psychological Care of Infant and Child* (1928), Watson advised parents, if they wanted the best results, to show no affection for their offspring. He wrote:

> Treat them as though they were young adults. Dress them, bathe them with care and circumspection. Let your behavior always be objective and firm. Never hug and kiss them, never let them sit on your lap. If you must, kiss them once on the forehead when they say goodnight. Shake hands with them in the morning . . .

> Remember when you are tempted to pet your child, that mother love is a dangerous instrument. An instrument which may inflict a never-healing wound, a wound which may make infancy unhappy, adolescence a nightmare, an instrument which may wreck your adult son or daughter's vocational future and their chances for marital happiness.[9]

This advice from Dr. Watson is pure nonsense, of course. Yet, in his day he was enormously popular, and millions of copies of his book were sold. Mothers and fathers worked diligently to "condition" their children in the way recommended by this "half-baked hot dog."[10]

Then came the controversial Dr. Sigmund Freud, followed by the pediatrician Dr. Benjamin Spock, who won fame and fortune with his book *Common Sense Book of Baby and Child Care*, first published in 1946. Up to the present time, nearly fifty million copies of this book in thirty languages have been sold.

Although he later acknowledged that it was Freud who "formed the whole basis of *Baby and Child Care*," Spock was careful not to credit Freud in his book. At the time, Freud was too controversial. His name alone evoked shudders.[11] Instead, Spock distilled Freudian theory into friendly phrases and American colloquialisms, and masked Freud's psychosexual stages of a child's development as the acquired wisdom of a Yankee country doctor.[12] Unknowingly, millions of parents who found Freud's theories totally unacceptable thus raised their beloved children according to his theories.

The essential message, articulated over and over again in the 1946 edition of *Baby and Child Care*, was twofold: parents should

not be alarmed at the expression of sexual and aggressive behavior—
it was natural. And, rather than interfering with their child's instinctual behavior, parents should become sensitive to the child's
instinctual needs.[13] In essence, Spock's message to parents was one
of permissiveness, promoting instant gratification and deviance. In
the 1960s, when the first generation "brought up on Spock" turned
into draft-dodging, free-loving hippies, conservatives rightly began
to blame the celebrated baby doctor.

Recently, shortly before his death, Benjamin Spock apologized
and said he had been wrong; his theories about raising children had
been hypotheses that did not bear out. In practice, healthy, responsible adults were not the outcome. It is good that he acknowledged
his mistake, but what about the millions who were duped believing
what he said?

By the 1950s, Spock had a whole bunch of followers, who
added fuel to the well-established fire of permissiveness. One of
them was Dr. Luther Woodward, whose ideas are paraphrased in
Your Child from Two to Five:

> What do you do when your preschool child calls you a "big
> stinker" or threatens to flush you down the toilet. Do you
> scold . . . punish . . . or sensibly take it in your stride? Dr.
> Woodward recommends a positive policy of understanding
> as the best and fastest way to help a child outgrow this verbal
> violence. When parents fully realize that all little tots feel
> angry and destructive at times, they're better able to mini-
> mize these outbursts. Once the preschool child gets rid of
> his hostility, the desire to destroy is gone and instinctive
> feelings of love and affection have a chance to sprout and
> grow. Once the child is six or seven, parents can rightly let
> the child know that he is expected to be outgrowing being
> cheeky to his parents.[14]

In addition to his "prudent" advice, Woodward adds that parents have to strengthen themselves against unjust critique: "But this
policy takes a broad perspective and a lot of composure, especially
when friends and relatives voice disapproval and warn you that you
are bringing up a brat."[15]

Recommendations such as these of Dr. Woodward were typical
of the advice given to parents—especially American parents—in the
1950s. They encouraged parents to be passive during the formative
years of their children—precisely the time during which they should

be taught respect for authority.

Dr. Woodward's suggestion is based on the simplistic notion that children will develop sweet and loving attitudes if parents will permit and encourage their temper tantrums during childhood. According to the optimistic—but extremely naive—expectations of Dr. Woodward, the tot who has been calling his mother a "big stinker" for six or seven years can be expected to embrace her suddenly in love and dignity. That outcome is most improbable. Dr. Woodward's creative policy of understanding (which actually means one should stand and do nothing) offers a "one-way ticket to emotional and social disaster."[16]

Another brand of permissive advice offered to parents in the mid-twenties was that of A. S. Neill. In a widely published book entitled *Summerhill: A Radical Approach to Childrearing,* Neill stated that parents have no right to insist on obedience from their children. Attempts to make the youngsters obey are merely designed to satisfy the adult's desire for power. There is no excuse for imposing parental wishes on children. They must be free. Neill stressed the importance of withholding responsibility from the child. Children must not be asked to work at all until they reach eighteen years. Parents should not even require them to help with small errands or assist with the chores. We insult them by making them do our menial tasks. Children should also not be required to say "thank you" or "please" to their parents. They should not even be *encouraged* to do so.[17]

By 1970, Neill's book had inexplicably sold over two million copies, primarily to schools of education in colleges and universities, where it was frequently a required text for student teachers.[18]

A more recent, and perhaps the most influential advisor of parents in America, is Dr. Thomas Gordon, a clinical psychologist. His program, *Parent Effectiveness Training* (PET) had gained so much recognition in the 1970s that *The New York Times* described it as "a national movement." More than one million copies of the first PET book were sold and nearly eight thousand PET classes were in operation throughout the country by 1976. Some churches have sponsored the training sessions for their laymen.[19]

In his program Dr. Gordon rejects parental authority in any form. Consider the following quotations from his first PET book:

> The stubborn persistence of the idea that parents must and should use authority in dealing with children has, in my opinion, prevented for centuries significant change or im-

provement in the way children are raised by parents and treated by adults (p. 168). Children resent those who have power over them (p. 177). Children do not want the parent to try to limit or modify their behavior by using or threatening to use authority. In short, children want to limit their behavior *themselves,* if it becomes apparent to *them* that their behavior must be limited or modified. Children, like adults, prefer to be their own authority over their behavior (p. 188). My own conviction is that as more people begin to understand power and authority more completely and accept its use as unethical, more parents . . . will be forced to search for creative new non-power methods that all adults can use with children and youth (p. 191).[20]

The sequel, *PET in Action,* is no different from the original. Especially noteworthy is that it recommends the works of the radical A. S. Neill "very strongly."[21]

By now an armada of psychologists, psychiatrists, and pediatricians has jumped on the bandwagon, selling and proclaiming new and off-the-wall suggestions on child rearing in their consulting rooms, in books, magazines, on the radio, and on TV. Most of these views, however, were anti-authoritative, directly contrary to the teachings of Scripture, which have for centuries been the foundation for many of the Western traditions of child rearing. In the Bible, children are continually admonished to obey their parents. Proverbs 1:8, for example, states, "Listen, my son, to your father's instruction and do not forsake your mother's teaching."

Why is parental authority so vigorously commanded in the Bible? Is it simply catering to the whims of oppressive, power-hunger adults, as Dr. Gordon and Dr. Neill would have it? No, as Dr. James Dobson states so correctly, the leadership of parents plays a significant role in the development of a child. Without respect for leadership there is anarchy, chaos, and confusion for everyone concerned. By learning to yield to the loving authority (leadership) of his parents, a child learns to submit to other forms of authority which will confront him later in life. The way he sees his parents' leadership sets the tone for his eventual relationships with his teachers, school principal, police, and employers. And, above all, while yielding to the loving leadership of their parents, children are also learning to yield to the benevolent leadership of God himself.[22]

The second mistake made by Woodward, Gordon, and many other bandwagon riders, is that they have based their advice of child rearing on the theory that the development of the child is mainly a process of maturation, and that learning plays no more than a supporting role. Rousseau, the father of the maturation theory, assumed that there is a natural development on which we can rely and which will inevitably take place, provided that we can keep in check the "unnatural" influences of society.[23]

If the development of a child is a process of maturation, it means that parents need not teach their children very much, if anything. Why would they indeed, if everything the child is intended to become is already in him? Parents only have to be "understanding," because once the child has "outgrown" his negative behavior, "instinctive feelings of love and affection [will] have a chance to sprout and grow," as Woodward promised.

Nothing, however, is further from the truth. The stories of children raised by wild animals unquestionably show that there is *nothing that any human being knows, or can do, that he has not learned.* (This of course excludes natural body functions, such as breathing, as well as reflexes, such as the involuntary closing of the eye when an object approaches it). This is a characteristic which very clearly distinguishes man from the animals.

Man Is Dependent on Learning

"A bear does not have to learn to be a bear, he simply is one. A duck needs no lessons in duckmanship. And an ant leads a perfectly satisfactory life without any instruction from other ants."[24] Even when isolated from birth, animals usually retain clearly recognizable instincts. A cat that is raised among dogs, will still behave like a cat. He won't try to bite the postman. There are only a few exceptions, such as the lion cub who would not be able to hunt the wildebeest when raised in isolation, and the nightingale who would not be able to sing.

A human being, on the other hand, "must *learn* to be human" (our italics).[25] He enters this world very poorly equipped. The knowledge a child needs to become fully human is not dormant. The story of Victor, as well as that of Amala and Kamala, present examples of man's total dependence on the "unnatural" influences of society, especially on learning. Amala and Kamala did not walk on all fours because they suffered from a "wolf disorder." After human education had become available to her, Kamala increasingly learned to act like a human being. A child must *learn* to walk erect, to talk, to eat with a knife and fork, to catch a ball, to ride a bicycle, to swim, etc. The ability to master these skills does not fall from the sky. A child must also learn to sustain his attention, to listen when spoken to, to follow through on instructions, to control his behavior and sit still and remain in his seat when the situation so requires. These abilities also do not happen automatically. The same principle is applicable for qualities such as friendliness, thankfulness, honesty, truthfulness, unselfishness, and respect for authority. And, as the primary educators of our children, it is our job as parents to teach our children these abilities and qualities.

If it is true that a child suffers from a mental disorder when he cannot do something because he has not learned it yet, then there must be hundreds, or even thousands of other "disorders" or "syndromes" that adults suffer from that have so far gone undiscovered. A person who cannot speak French because he has not learned the language yet, would therefore suffer from a "French-speaking deficit disorder" (FSDD). Somebody who cannot play golf because he has not learned the game yet, suffers from a "golf-playing deficit disorder" (GPDD). And if somebody cannot play chess, he must be suffering from a "chess-playing deficit disorder" (CPDD).

The inability of psychology and psychiatry to take note of the fundamental characteristics of the human being, that there is nothing that any human being knows, or can do, that he has not learned, has made them popular with many parents. Their quick-fix solutions, involving labels around childrens' necks and drug prescriptions to make parents' lives easier, actually exempt parents from their responsibilities. Parents only have to be "understanding," because the drug will do the job for them (although, tragically, it never does). Equally tragically, many parents are happy to follow this route.

Then, there are parents who have become so obsessed with the idea that there is something wrong with their children that no amount of reasoning will convince them otherwise. We recently learned about a mother—she is also the president of a support group for parents with hyperactive children—who is spending her life trying to find the food and/or food additives that are responsible for her three "hyperactive" boys' poor behavior. While she is fanatically searching for the answer, the two elder boys, respectively eleven and eight, are physically assaulting each other and their three-year-old brother, and have even tried to set their thatched-roof house on fire. They set all their teddy bears alight, as well as lighting fires on the carpets. While shopping with their mother some time ago at a grocery store, they threw whatever they could lay their hands on at other customers. The youngest, it seems, has the habit of perching himself on the balcony of their three story home. Frankly, we would prefer not to be around when these boys reach puberty. We shudder to think what they will probably be like as adults.

On the other hand, there are millions of parents who are desperately in search of a solution to their children's problems. They want only the best for the children in their care. They are willing to take responsibility, to listen, and to learn. It is for these parents that this book offers a ray of hope. Contrary to most other books on child rearing, however, it does not put forward any new or outlandish theory, but depends on Biblical wisdom, truth and logic.

Notes

1. Schmidt, W. H. O., *Child Development: The Human, Cultural, and Educational Context* (New York: Harper & Row, 1973), 26-29.

2. Olivier, J. "Deur wolwe grootgemaak," Huisgenoot, 7 March, 126-127.

3. Schmidt, *Child Development*, 22.

4. Ibid., xv.

5. Ibid., 11-12.

6. Burrows, L., *Good Children* (London: Corgi Books, 1986), Introduction.

7. Ibid.

8. Dobson, J., *The New Dare to Discipline* (Wheaton, Illinois: Tyndale House Publishers, Inc., 1992), 17.

9. Watson, J. B., & Watson, R., *Psychological Care of Infant and Child* (London: Allen and Unwin, 1928), 73.

10. Dobson, *The New Dare to Discipline*, 73.

11. Maier, T., "The book on Dr. Spock," *Newsday*, 18 March 1998, B03.

12. Walton, D., "You probably know less than you think about Dr. Spock," *Minneapolis Star Tribune*, 3 May 1998.

13. Kramer, Y., "Freud and the culture wars: Part 3," *The Public Interest*, 1 June 1996.

14. Woodward, L., Edwards, M. (ed.), *Your Child from Two to Five* (New York: Permabooks, 1955), 95-96.

15. Ibid.

16. Dobson, J., *The Strong-Willed Child* (Eastbourne: Kingsway Publications, 1993), 54.

17. Dobson, J., *Dare to Discipline* (Toronto: Bantam Books, 1977), 92-94.

18. Eakman, B. K., *Cloning of the American Mind: Eradicating Morality through Education* (Lafayette: Huntington House Publishers, 1998), 112.

19. Gordon, T., *P.E.T. in Action* (Toronto: Bantam Books, 1976.), 1.

20. Gordon, T., *Parent Effectiveness Training* (New York: David McKay Company, Inc., 1970), 164, 177, 188, 191.

21. Gordon, *P.E.T. in Action*, 358.

22. Dobson, *The Strong-Willed Child*, 164-165.

23. Schmidt, *Child Development*, 5-6.

24. McKern, S. S., *The Many Faces of Man* (New York: Lothrop, Lee & Shephard Co., 1972).

25. Ibid.

5.

Questions Most Frequently Asked

When confronted with the information in the first four chapters, the four questions listed below are raised almost automatically. As they will shed more light on our topic of discussion, we have included these questions with their appropriate answers.

Q *You have called ADHD a myth. That implies that an armada of psychiatrists, psychologists and medical specialists are wrong. But why would they continue to proclaim ideas that are unproven, and why would they prescribe harmful medication?*

A The popularity of an idea does not give it any scientific validity. Before it was proved that the earth is round, everybody believed it to be flat. The popularity of the idea did not make it true. Science, therefore, does not always "advance by consensus," as is maintained by Galaburda.[1]

One explanation for the fact that many experts continue to cling to this obvious myth, is that of *ignorance*. This is what they have been taught at university, and they simply accept it as the truth. But the "truth" they have been taught may not be true at all. The human sciences are certainly not exact sciences, and therefore it happens quite easily that they run off the rails. As Popkin and Stroll remarked in 1969, "The history of science is replete with theories that have been thoroughly believed by the wisest men and were then thoroughly discredited."[2] This saying aptly describes the present situation.

Secondly, ADHD and all the other so-called mental diseases have become money-makers for both mental health professions and mental health centers. By continually creating new psychiatric categories of disease (such as ADHD) and subsequently ascribing diagnostic codes to them in the DSM, health specialists and services can claim from insurance benefits or medical aids for more and more people for more and more diseases. It seems that, in many cases, money is the only consideration:

> Psychiatric admissions for children and adolescents to private hospitals tripled between 1980 and 1986. Irving Phillips, professor of psychiatry at the University of California, San Francisco, School of Medicine, pointed out that "Excessive hospitalization of troubled young people has been a problem for some time, but has increased in the 1980s." Congressional hearings published in 1992 under the title "How Psychiatric Treatment Bilks the System and Betrays Our Trust," were told of children kept in for-profit hospitals for periods determined not by medical needs, but duration of insurance benefits, as well as bounties paid for referrals to school, emergency room, and law enforcement personnel and even to clergy. Psychiatrist Walter Afield testified that, according to "The DSM III . . . everyone in this room will fit into two or three of the diagnoses. . . . Every new disease . . . gets a new hospital program, new admissions, a new system, and a way to bilk it."[3]

Psychiatrist Ron Leifer concurs. Scoffing at the tendency in his field to find mental illness in everything, he said:

> Everyone is neurotic. I have no trouble giving out diagnoses. In my office, I see only abnormal people. Out of my office, I see only normal people. It's up to me. It's just a joke. This is what I mean by this fraud, this arrogant fraud. . . . To make some kind of pretension that this is a scientific statement is . . . damaging to the culture. . . . [T]he more popular psychiatry becomes, the more mentally ill people there are. This is good business.[4]

Not only is it "good business" for the mental health professions and mental health centers, but in the United States also for low-income families and schools. Isn't it amazing, that even parents can nowadays be rewarded for watching and even helping life's most precious stones go down the drain.

> In 1990, the doors were opened to a lucrative cash welfare program to low-income parents whose children were diagnosed with ADHD. A family could get more than $450 a month for each ADHD child. The impact was telling. In 1989, children citing mental impairment that included ADHD, made up only 5 percent of all disabled kids on the

program. That figure rose to nearly 25 percent by 1995. To obtain the payout, some parents actually coached their children to do poorly in school and to act weird.

In 1991, eligibility rules changed for federal educational grants, providing schools with $400 in annual grant money for each child diagnosed with ADHD. The same year, the Department of Education formally recognized ADHD as a handicap and directed all state education officers to establish procedures to screen and identify ADHD children and provide them with special educational and psychological services.

Dr. Fred A. Baughman, Jr., a California pediatric neurologist, says that the frequency with which learning disorders and ADHD are diagnosed in schools "is proportional to the presence and influence within the schools of mind/brain behavioral diagnosticians, testers, and therapists."

Today, American schools spend a combined $1 billion a year on psychologists who work full-time to diagnose students. As of 1996, $15 billion was being spent annually in the U.S. on the diagnosis, treatment and study of these so-called "disorders."[5]

Of course a beneficiary in the ADHD money-chain not to be overlooked is the pharmaceutical industry, whose profits depend on the continuation of this myth. According to IMS America, a company which tracks drug sales, sales of Ritalin have increased from $109 million in 1992 to $336 million in 1996.[6]

The only people involved in this myth who do not seem to benefit in any way are the children who are labeled and have to live with the stigma for the rest of their lives. In fact, as previous chapters have shown, this "disease" can cause tremendous suffering in the short term, and have dreadful outcomes in the long term.

If you find it hard to accept that mammon can become the only consideration despite the consequences, ponder the still widely used psychiatric practice of electroshock (also known as "electroconvulsive therapy" or ECT). ECT was introduced by psychiatrist Ugo Cerletti. He visited a slaughterhouse in Rome in the late 1930s where operators used electric shock to send pigs into epileptic convulsions in order to make it easier to slit their throats.[7] Shortly thereafter he started using electroshock on humans. Toward the end of his life, as he recalled the first time that he had tried ECT on a human being, Cerletti remarked to a colleague: "When I saw the patient's reaction, I thought to myself: This ought to be abolished!"[8]

During ECT, a rubber gag is placed to stop the patient from breaking his teeth or biting his tongue. The electrodes are placed on the temples. A button is pushed and between one hundred and two hundred volts of electricity send a current searing through the temples or from the front to the back of the head. This creates a severe convulsion or seizure of long duration, called a "grand mal" convulsion, which is identical to an epileptic fit. The entire procedure takes between five and fifteen minutes. Most patients are given a total of six to twelve shocks, one a day, three times a week. Most patients are given more than one series of treatments.[9]

Shock treatment during the 1940s and 1950s was a very raw affair. Convulsions were so violent, broken bones were common, particularly in the spine. One researcher, for example, X-rayed every patient after his or her first course of shock treatment and discovered that 20 percent had compression fractures of the vertebrae. To remedy this problem and the general unpleasantness of patients thrashing about during ECT, psychiatrists began using muscle relaxants and anesthesia. Thus, electroshock in the 1960s was redefined as "modified ECT." Of course, the use of muscle relaxants and anesthesia caused the body to lie still, but did not reduce the impact the shock had on the brain and nervous system. If anything, *more* current was now needed to bring about a convulsion.[10]

The literature continued to depict the destructive effects of ECT: brain damage, memory lapses and disturbances, loss of bowel and bladder control, delirium, delusions, hallucinations, damage to the spine, clavicle and femur, and even death. A 1993 study involving the elderly concluded: "27 percent of shock patients were dead within one year compared with 4 percent of a similar group treated with antidepressant drugs. In two years, 46 percent of shocked patients were dead vs. 10 percent who had the drugs."[11] In Texas, 6 out of 1,656 people in 1994 were reported to have died within fourteen days of ECT, a death rate of 0.36. The same percentage makes up the *combined* death rate for cancer, stroke, lung disease, motor vehicle accidents, diabetes, HIV infection, suicide, liver disease (and cirrhosis), and homicide in 1994.[12] Despite these and many other damaging conclusions reached by researchers, ECT is portrayed by psychiatrists as painless, safe, and effective.

"Electroshock is done by psychiatrists who give it for a living," says Dr. Michael Chavin, "and therefore have a financial incentive in saying that it is harmless."[13] In fact, the financial incentive is quite substantial. The income from this "harmless" procedure for the psychiatric industry in the U.S. alone makes an estimated three billion dollars per year.[14]

Q *If ADHD does not have a biological cause, why does this problem, according to statistics, tend to run in families?*

A The implication of the question is that ADHD is passed on genetically. One should never lose sight of the fact, however, that statistical evidence is often no more than circumstantial in nature. Circumstantial evidence must always be interpreted. Unfortunately it can easily be misinterpreted.

It may be useful to present an example of how unwise it can be to base conclusions on statistics only. Until recently, the inhabitants of some towns in South Africa were allowed to use well water for domestic purposes. In some of these places, the water, when used as drinking water, caused a discoloring of the front teeth. Except in the case of a person with dentures, all the members of the family—father, mother and children—would then have discolored front teeth. The concordance must have been 100 percent. As already indicated, however, the discoloring of the teeth was not caused by genetics, but by the circumstances which the family shared (i.e., that they all drank the same water).

Another example of the circumstantial nature of statistics is the fact that children raised by English-speaking parents speak English, children raised by Spanish-speaking parents speak Spanish, and children raised by French-speaking parents speak French. Except for exceptional cases where children do not learn to speak at all, the concordance would be 100 percent. Surely nobody would attribute this fact to heredity, but to the fact that a child learns to speak the language (or sometimes languages) which he hears on a daily basis.

It should be noted that, unless they speak to him in Spanish, the child of the English-speaking parents will not be able to speak Spanish, not because there is anything wrong with him, but simply because his parents did not teach him to speak Spanish. The inability to speak Spanish will also run in the family, but is certainly not genetic.

The fact that ADHD often runs in families can therefore not be attributed to genetics, but can be caused by the fact that the family members share the same unique environment. Of course such problems can also be the result of learning, or the lack of it.

Q *I can accept that the ADHD notion has been blown out of proportion. But surely there must be some children, even if the number is minuscule, whose behavior problems are genuinely caused by biological factors and who would therefore benefit from drugs?*

A Of course there might be cases where biological factors contribute to behavior problems. Even if this is the case, it neither implies that a child suffers from a mental illness, nor does it warrant the use of drugs. A comparison to a physical condition should make this clear.

Susan's (the coauthor's) elder son, Gustav, was born very small and thin, and he walked with a clumsy gait with one leg bent inwards at an awkward angle. As many other parents hope for their children with ADHD, she and her husband also hoped that he would eventually outgrow his problem. He did not. At the age of seven, although he had been somewhat involved in sports since the age of four, his physical condition was still unchanged.

About a year and a half ago, Susan and her husband decided to take action. Gustav was very keen on playing hockey, and soon after the decision had been made, he was practicing ice hockey and roller hockey rigorously at least three times per week. In less than a year, his physical appearance was as normal as that of any other child of his height and his leg was no longer a source of concern. In fact, not only has his body improved, and is still improving, but he is in very good health and has developed exceptional self-esteem.

Without doubt, Gustav's condition was genuinely caused by biological factors. However, we are convinced that people would have raised their eyebrows if Susan and her husband had turned to anabolic steroids to improve his physical appearance. The negative effects of steroids outweigh their positive effects, in the same way that the negative effects of stimulants outweigh their positive effects. There is a place for medicine, and it should never be kept from a child if he should need it. However, there are limits to its use. Although stimulants might offer a temporary relief to some children's behavioral and learning problems, one should always consider the long-term effects. These, unfortunately, are very poor indeed. The true solution for these children's problems, although it requires some commitment and effort, is not temporary, but lasting.

Q *If the role of a parent is so overwhelmingly important, why do our three children differ so enormously from each other, when the same parents, in the same environment, have raised them in exactly the same way? Surely you cannot deny that biological factors, such as genes, play an important role in the development of a child's personality, behavior and abilities?*

A We are not denying that a person's genes or his heredity play a role in lending him his uniqueness. In fact, studies of identical twins that were separated soon after birth and later brought together again, indicate that heredity certainly does play a role. The history of such studies abounds with stories that seem to reveal such twins as "two halves of the same self." Although they were raised by different families, they fell down stairs at the same age, got married and miscarried in the same year, seemingly communicated "telepathically" across thousands of miles, while "evil" twins even committed arson or murder at about the same time. Many of these twins had similar personality traits when they were reunited. And yet, the lives of identical twins, even those raised by the same parents, are full of just as many instances of discordance, differences and disaffection.[15]

Although heredity plays a role, it is not as overwhelmingly important as we have been given to believe by psychiatry and psychology. Neither is the environment, another factor frequently presented as *the* determinant of personality, behavior and abilities. The point is that psychiatry and psychology have overlooked one important factor, and that is the role of *education*. Obviously Amala's and Kamala's heredity had nothing to do with their wolflike behavior. Their behavior was also not a result of the environment they had shared. That would imply that, should we have raised our own children in the same forest, they would also have acted like wolves. We sincerely doubt this. The only logical explanation for their wolflike behavior can be the *lack of human education* they had experienced.

Human life can be compared to a game of cards. At birth, every person is dealt a hand of cards—his genetic makeup. Some receive a good hand, others a less good one. The outcome of the game of life, however, is not solely determined by the quality of a person's initial hand of cards, but also by the way in which he takes part in the game of life. The quality of a person's participation in the game of life does not depend only on heredity, but also on the environment and especially on the education he received as a child. Parents, as the primary educators of their children, have a greater role to play than anything or anybody else in the way their children will take part in the game of life, both while they are children and also, eventually when they are adults. Of course, apart from heredity, environment, and education, there may be other factors—so far undiscovered—that also play a role in determining the uniqueness of every person.

We have to reject the suggestion in the question under discussion that parents can raise two children in exactly the same way. This is simply not possible, since it would imply that a parent has to literally duplicate everything he has said to and done with the first child to and with the second. Even if this could be possible—and it definitely is not—it would be a grave mistake, because education should always be provided according to *individual needs*.

All human beings have the physical need to eat, but the quantity of this need can differ considerably from one person to the next. Johnny and Peter may be more or less the same age and size, but when Mommy serves them dinner, Johnny's plate is always fuller than Peter's. Children differ in more ways than just the amount of food that they consume. Johnny may be a docile, generous and peaceful person, and therefore relatively easy to raise. Peter, on the other hand, may be prone to defiance, selfishness, hostility, and uncontrollable behavior. Although we agree that the differences between the two brothers can be neurologically determined, we are doubtful whether such neurological differences represent "disorders" or "syndromes." These differences do not imply that Peter has ADHD, ODD, or CD, but simply mean that Daddy and Mommy are going to have to work harder to equip Peter with the right attitudes and to shape him into becoming a respectful and responsible citizen.

Parenthood is a skill, and just as all other human skills, it must also be learned. The problem is that parents of today, due to the interruption of the child-rearing traditions, do not have the *knowledge* to raise children in general, let alone raise children such as Peter. Without proper knowledge, parents are unable to intervene in their children's lives. Even with good intentions at heart, they can, at best, stand passively and watch how their children determine their own futures. All too often, parents must watch their children self-destruct.

As stated above, the knowledge needed to raise children was traditionally passed on from generation to generation. Although these child-rearing traditions certainly had their shortcomings, they were, contrary to the ridiculous and outlandish advice invented by American psychologists and psychiatrists today, many times more successful in producing balanced, educated, and well-behaved children, and eventually turning these children into responsible adults.

Notes

1. Galaburda, A. M., "Learning Disability: Biological, societal, or both? A response to Gerald Coles," *Journal of Learning Disabilities*, vol. 22(5), 1989, 278-282.

2. Popkin, R. H., & Stroll, A., *Philosophy Made Simple* (London: WH Allen, 1969), 167.

3. Baughman, F. A, Jr., "The future of mental health: Radical changes ahead," *USA Today*, vol. 125, 1 March 1997, 60.

4. Eakman, B. K., *Cloning of the American Mind: Eradicating Morality through Education* (Lafayette, LA: Huntington House Publishers, 1998), 96.

5. "Witch doctors, shamans. The birth of the 'cult' of child psychology," *Psychiatry: Betraying and Drugging Children* (Los Angeles: CCHR, 1998), 8-11.

6. Russell, J., "The pill that teachers push," *Good Housekeeping*, vol. 225, 1 December 1997.

7. Röder, T., Kubillus, V., & Burwell, A., *Psychiatrists: The Men Behind Hitler* (Los Angeles: Freedom Publishing, 1994), 206.

8. Szasz, T., *The Manufacture of Madness* (New York: Harper & Row, 1970), 31.

9. "Perpetuating cruelty," *Psychiatry Destroys Minds* (Los Angeles: CCHR, 1997), 6-9.

10. Wiseman, B., *Psychiatry: The Ultimate Betrayal* (Los Angeles: Freedom Publishing, 1995), 119, 122.

11. Kroesser, D., & Fogel, B. S., "Electroconvulsive therapy for major depression in the oldest old," *The American Journal of Geriatric Psychiatry*, vol. 1(1), 1993.

12. "Unsafe and ineffective," *Psychiatry Destroys Minds* (Los Angeles: CCHR, 1997), 24-27.

13. "What psychiatrists say about electroshock," *Psychiatry Destroys Minds* (Los Angeles: CCHR, 1997), 32-35.

14. Ibid.

15. Neimark, J., Cochran, T., & Dossey, L., "Nature's clones," *Psychology Today*, vol. 30, 1 July 1997.

6.

The Decomposition of Society

On the first day of an elementary psychology course at Johns Hopkins University [in the 1950s], a professor sat on his desk silently reading the morning newspaper. The bell rang, but he didn't seem to notice it. Then audibly he began to read the headlines of the front page articles. They captioned difficult world problems, spoke of inhuman acts of man to his fellow man, and, in general, painted the typical sensational front page picture one may read every day. Presently, he looked up and said, "The world is in a mess." He spent the rest of the hour explaining how psychology is the world's one hope for straightening out that mess.[1]

Yet, despite the fact that psychology and psychiatry have succeeded in entering our schools, our courts, our legislatures, our workplaces, and, bit by bit, our homes, the newspaper headlines have not improved. They continue to report about lawlessness and greed, an increase in youth violence, robberies, theft and deceit, overcrowded prisons, a decay of morality, child abuse, alcoholism, a growing drug industry and usage, the disintegration of the family, an increase in teenage pregnancies and teen suicide, a lack of motivation from students, an ever-declining literacy rate, dwindling test scores, and graduates who can't even find their home city on a map. In short, the world is in a far greater mess than what it was imagined to be in during the 1950s, and probably has ever been in before.

Although many things have changed since the 1950s, the greatest difference between then and today is that the mid-twentieth century was still characterized by certainties and security, while the present time is not. In our increasingly competitive and technical society, with science assuming more and more influence in our daily lives, complexity and the accelerating speed of change have been accepted as an intrinsic part of existence. Imitating science, today we have become a society that thirsts for change, for new ideas, for the latest model, for the fastest and easiest way. We have become a society of instant coffee, instant replays and instant gratification.[2]

Just as today's computer becomes tomorrow's trade-in, with the inexorable advance of technology, the cultural norms and expectancies which characterized our society for centuries have undergone drastic transformation. While no one would argue against change for the better, mankind survives best in a predictable and ordered environment where change is capable of being understood and managed. This, however, is not the kind of transformation we have seen in Western society.[3]

As Clem Sunter points out, children growing up in the 1950s still had a narrow definition of family and gender roles and a sharp perception of social class. Children were accustomed to two parents, with perhaps one or two sisters or brothers. The mother stayed at home while father went off to work. If children did something wrong, they were disciplined. At school, a hierarchy existed where students accepted teachers as their superiors.[4] Today, on the contrary, traditional families are labeled as "straight families," one of many kinds of "family units." Sex without moderation is promoted as a way of life. Now, children are surprised if they have a mother and a father to bring them up. More than likely, they will never meet their fathers, who, in any case, never support them. The word "bastard" has lost its significance. Should they have two parents, they almost expect both of them to be pursuing careers at the same time.

At one time, sending children to school meant a guarantee of a structured, nurturing, and effective education; today parents are concerned about the failure of modern education—declining moral standards and escalating drug abuse, crime, and violence in schools. Parents rightly worry that they are less and less in control of—or relevant to—the direction that their children's education takes. The children, on the other hand, soon learn that teachers are their equals and can at any time be treated with disdain.[5]

When leaving school before and during the 1950s, a youngster would repeat the process he had become accustomed to as a child. A man knew that he would get a job, get married, and have children. Today, however, there is no certainty of a job and being on welfare is a pleasant alternative. If they're like their parents, they'll take Prozac or Valium and chant "don't worry, be happy."[6]

Where once citizens understood that justice existed to protect the innocent, the public is now expected to be sympathetic to the supposed "insanities" suffered by mass murderers, child abusers, sexual deviants, and other criminals.[7]

According to the "best" minds, virtues and even the basic concepts of right and wrong can no longer be considered the foundation of an ordered society. Instead, they are supposedly the causes of individual stress, guilt, and many more of our social ills. Children are being taught that they are their own authority on questions of morals and values with no reference to fundamental ethical precepts that have been the driving force of civilization for centuries.[8] Today, everyone has a right to his own opinion and his own way of life, even though these opinions are often without knowledge, and this way of life harms, abuses, or destroys others and himself in the process.

Religion once retained a pervasive and guiding moral influence, and the neighborhood was a community with norms and good neighborliness.[9] Subjected to the same forces of change as the rest of society, religion itself is now widely criticized and even attacked by authority as outmoded, irrelevant, unscientific, and thereby ill-equipped to address the problems and stresses of modern society. As U.S. Supreme Court Justice Antonin Scalia recently observed, our so-called worldly-wise society has become openly hostile to religious believers, scoffing at traditions and beliefs.[10]

In other words, there are no guarantees about anything. So now, according to Sunter, we have authority gaps and ethics gaps:

> This may sound like a new version of the old generation gap, but it isn't. Certainly the 1920s . . . and the 1950s and the 1960s had rebels . . . and angry young men. But at least in those days there was a structure and an establishment. Today there is no structure because everything is relative. Even the Ten Commandments are up for grabs. "Thou shalt not kill" has become "thou shalt kill under certain circumstances and let's negotiate the circumstances." Without absolute moral truths, the younger generation have no navigational aids. Without the wrath of an Old Testament God, they have no fear of retribution. Even Hell is no longer pictured as a place of eternal torment, a flaming pit full of demons and devils. Fire and brimstone have been replaced by a "state of nonbeing." Add to this the absence of authority and hierarchy in this world and you have no checks on youthful behavior at all.[11]

If you believe that this is a bit heavy, take a good look at the list of the top disciplinary problems in U.S. schools in 1940 compared to 1990. The source was not a right-wing organization, but the *Congressional Quarterly*, November 1993. The list on the left consists of minor infractions whereas the list on the right is about major criminal activity:

1940	1990
Talking out of turn	Drug abuse
Chewing gum	Alcohol abuse
Making a noise	Sexual behavior
Running in hallways	(Attempted) suicide
Queue-jumping	Rape, sexual assault
Ignoring dress code	Robbery, theft
Litter	Physical assault

Merely listing them, however, does not provide one with a full understanding of the magnitude of these problems. It is therefore important to further elaborate on the alarming manifestation of each of these criminal activities in our present society.

Apart from these activities, an issue that cannot be ignored is the matter of literacy. If the above-mentioned activities are the problems faced by schools today, what then, has happened to literacy— once the heart and soul of the educational institution?

Youth, Violence, and Delinquency—Our Social Toxin

The 82-year-old Los Angeles grandmother recently was killed on the porch of her Watts neighborhood home by a stray bullet. It was fired by a gang of boys who had just kidnapped, tortured and raped a 13-year-old girl in the abandoned building next door. When a suspect described by police as "dangerous and violent" turned himself in, accompanied by his mother, he turned out to be a kid who had just turned 12, two days after the crime.[12]

Bomb squads yesterday searched for booby traps in a high school where two teenage gunmen killed at least 13 people before turning the guns on themselves in the worst mass shooting in the U.S. . . . Police said 20 others were critically injured in the shooting spree. . . . Before Tuesday, the worst school shooting in the United States took place in March last year in Jonesboro, Arkansas, when two boys, aged 11 and 13, shot and killed a teacher and four girls. That was one of a series of incidents at U.S. schools in which at least 14 people were killed and more than 40 wounded in less than two years.[13]

They pillaged and plundered, sparing little at Sunny Hills High School. Besides the 100 shattered windows, battered computers and ransacked classrooms, they also went after the heart of the Fullerton school, damaging a 25-year-old athletic trophy, old photos, and other mementos.

That was in January. A month later, at a different campus, a different squad of invaders smashed lights and splattered paint through the halls of La Puente High School. Then they desecrated the senior wall, drenching the mounted names of graduating seniors with paint and gouging the school's 36-year-old mosaic insignia.[14]

Even in a tranquil, rural community in Texas, 11 children between the ages of 8 and 14 clubbed a quarter horse to death, and some of them laughed and boasted when police arrested them at school.[15]

Although most people never get used to them, motiveless and senseless crimes such as the above have become a common phenomenon in modern Western society. This was not always the case. In his 1983 *Encyclopedia of Mass Murder*, Colin Wilson reports, "We call a crime motiveless if it seems to do no one any good. Before 1960 such crimes were rare, and the few that occurred belong to the end of the decade."[16] Focusing on the youth, Los Angeles County Attorney Gil Garcetti remarked on the same phenomenon in 1994. "It's incredible," he said, "the ability of the very young to commit the most horrendous crimes imaginable and not have a second thought about it. This was unthinkable twenty years ago."[17]

Since 1960, the violent crime rate in America has increased at least fivefold. In 1960, there were 160.9 violent crimes per one hundred thousand citizens; in 1992 there were 757.5.[18] The second figure is alarming, not only due to the tremendous increase in crime it represents, but especially due to the ages of the offenders it includes. Juvenile delinquency once meant speeding in hod rods. Today, children kill other children without compunction or remorse. Even ten years ago, defendants in homicide cases averaged between ages twenty and twenty-five. Now defendants are typically aged fifteen to twenty.[19]

Police records of violent youth show that arrests of young Americans between the ages of thirteen and twenty for homicide, robbery, and aggravated assault increased greatly in the 1960s (as much as 84 percent in the case of homicide). During the following decade, arrests for persons under eighteen years of age for eight serious crimes increased more than 231 percent. In 1981, juveniles accounted for over one out of three arrests for robbery, one out of every three arrests for crime against property, one out of six arrests for rape, and one out of eleven arrests for murder. In 1981, about one teenager out of every fifteen in the nation was arrested.[20] Between 1983 and 1991, crimes committed by juveniles under eighteen showed another staggering increase: robberies have increased five times, murders have tripled, and rapes have doubled.[21] More than five hundred children arrested for rape in 1991 were under twelve.[22]

Schools are no longer the safe havens they once were—places where students were free to develop and learn the skills necessary to have successful, productive lives. During the 1996-1997 academic year, 6,093 students were expelled for bringing firearms or explosives to school. A recent study by the U.S. Department of Justice and the National Association of School Psychologists provides startling figures: every day 100,000 children take guns to schools. Each day 6,250 teachers are threatened and 260 teachers are assaulted. Some 14,000 young people are attacked on school property every day, and 160,000 children miss school every day because of the fear of violence. A large percentage of these at-risk, antisocial children are vulnerable to gang recruitment and membership. Being a gang member is strongly associated with an increase in violent behavior and greatly increases the chances of one's being victimized by violence. Gang membership in the United States is now estimated at 650,000. Ominously, the all-girl gang has been the fastest growing sector of the gang culture in the United States in recent years.

Cold-bloodedness has become commonplace. "Youngsters used to shoot each other in the body. Then in the head," Judge Susan R. Winfield said in 1994. "Now they shoot each other in the face."[23]

In Canada, the rate of violent crime doubled in the 1960s, increased by 30 percent in the 1970s and rose another 46 percent in the 1980s.[24] The Ontario Teachers' Federation reported that major incidents of violence in the schools increased 150 percent between 1987 and 1990. In 1991, young offenders in Canada were charged with double the violent offences (18,000) compared with 1986 figures (9,300). The Manitoba Teachers' Society said that one in ten teachers reported physical attacks between September 1991 and January 1993. Authorities were reluctant to see this as a wave of violence, but students pointed out that a lot of other incidents are not reported.[25]

While the reported violent crime rate for Canadian boys has leveled off since 1991, it is still 85 percent higher than a decade ago, and the rate for girls is growing. The number of girls charged with violent criminal offences increased 179 percent between 1987 and 1997. In the same period, robbery rates for girls increased 417 percent and for boys 166 percent.[26]

Statistics, however, cannot depict the pain and fear that result from the true-life tragedies they reflect. In May 1998, Tom Pham, a 17-year-old twelfth grade student in Toronto, was murdered. A 14-year-old ninth grade student from another school in the area was charged with second-degree murder in Tom's death from multiple stab wounds at a local snack bar. Students and staff from both schools were horrified. The schools might be safe, but after the incident, students said they no longer make eye contact with some people between school and home in case they take offense. As one student said, "When I take the subway, I sort of put my head down and don't look at anybody . . . you never know, they might have a gun or a knife."[27]

In Britain, although the number of homicides per year has remained unchanged since 1857—thirteen per million of the population[28]—the total rate of violent crimes against individuals has increased a frightening 1,200 percent between 1960 and 1993. The number of robberies has increased by 2,700 percent in the same period.[29] At present, 93 percent of Britain's crime—more than five million recorded indictable offences per year—is against property. That is a great many, and there are an estimated three times more unreported. In fact, it is terrifying if one compares it to the figure of 1918 when there were only 80,000 reported offenses.[30]

Between 1991 and 1996, female violent crime in Britain has risen by 12 percent, four times the rate among men, and offenses involving women carrying out assault, robbery, murder and drug-related crimes have increased by 250 percent since 1973. Although the numbers remain small, with 9,500 women found guilty of violence against another person in 1994, compared to 5,300 in 1984, a clear pattern is emerging: women are becoming more violent.[31]

Most disturbing are the signs of increased violence among younger women who, at the most extreme level, are forming menacing American-style gangs in some inner-city housing projects. In one survey, it emerged that in the fifteen to seventeen age group, girls are more likely to take pleasure in violence than boys are. Kidscape, a child protection charity, has seen an increase in the number of calls from girls who are the victims of violent attacks by other girls. The charity received 80 reports of violence in 1993, which rose to 97 in 1994 and to 119 in 1995, varying from kicking and pushing to one group attack in which a girl was pinned down in the showers by classmates who pushed a bar of soap into her anus.[32]

Although the total number of reported crimes in France has fallen slightly in recent years, juvenile delinquency has continued to rise sharply—by 81 percent over the past ten years, according to the Ministry of the Interior. One in five of those charged is now under eighteen, the age of criminal responsibility, twice the proportion of twenty-five years ago. Gangs of 8-year-olds are no longer unusual. And only one juvenile delinquent in ten, it is reckoned, gets caught.

"Every day new limits are being broken, beyond which society begins to fall apart," said President Jacques Chirac in his 1997 New Year's Eve message. A few hours later, gangs of youths, most of them aged twelve to sixteen, went on a rampage in Strasbourg, leaving sixty burnt-out cars, thirty broken bus shelters and four vandalized municipal buildings—just for the hell of it, apparently. No one was killed; only two people were injured; little appears to have been stolen. But the riot confirmed the belief that urban youth violence has reached unprecedented proportions.

Strasbourg was far from an isolated case. Hardly a week goes by without some new outbreak of unrest. Attacks on bus and metro drivers (up by more than 50 percent in two years) prompted public-transport strikes in eighteen big towns in November 1997. Teachers have been protesting against the spread of pupil violence, now affecting half of all secondary schools.[33]

Other Western countries' crime rates parallel the trend of the United States, Canada, Britain, and France. In Australia, the number of serious assaults, for example, has risen 391 percent between 1973-74 and 1991-92, and the robbery rate increased 190 percent.[34] In New Zealand, the total number of violent offences increased 615 percent between 1960 and 1990, from 2,937 to 20,987.[35] The crime rate in Greece has increased 1,268 percent between 1980 and 1990.[36]

In Sweden, the per-capita crime has gone up fivefold since 1950,[37] and in Germany the number of arrests for robberies has increased 60 percent between 1972 and 1985. Assault and theft rose 71 percent.[38] In 1993, a murder was committed every three hours.[39] In only one year, in 1997, the number of crimes committed by German children up to age fourteen surged 10.1 percent to about 144,000 cases. Crimes committed by young people between fourteen and eighteen years of age rose by 5.4 percent.[40]

As already indicated, children with so-called ADHD are especially at risk of becoming involved in criminal activities. Well-controlled studies of children with ADHD find that at least 70 percent continue to meet the full diagnostic criteria for the disorder into adolescence. By young adulthood, this population has more academic problems and is more oppositional and delinquent than peer groups. Compared to other young adults, they, according to Mannuzza et al., engage in activities that result in more school suspension (14 percent v. 2 percent), have more adversarial contacts with law enforcement agencies (19:3), and are more likely to be admitted into juvenile justice facilities (5:1).[41]

One study, published in 1989, followed 103 males in New York State who had been diagnosed with ADHD at ages ranging from six to twelve. When this group reached sixteen to twenty-three years, the team conducted follow-up interviews with the subjects and their parents. The researchers then compared the subjects' arrest records with a control group of one hundred individuals in the same age range. The researchers found that significantly higher percentages of individuals with ADHD had been arrested (39 percent v. 20 percent), convicted of a crime (28:11), and incarcerated (9:1).[42]

The Frightening Drug Scene

According to police, much of the violence is related to drug abuse. This is confirmed by research. A study released in 1989 indicated that more than half of those arrested for serious crimes in fourteen American cities who volunteered for drug testing were, in fact, drug users. In Philadelphia, the figure was 82 percent.[43]

A comprehensive survey of self-reported offenses among a representative sample of over five thousand secondary students in New South Wales, Australia, revealed that nearly half of NSW secondary students reported that they had participated in some form of crime in the last twelve months: 29 percent of students had assaulted someone; 27 percent had maliciously damaged property; 15 percent had received or sold stolen goods; 9 percent had shoplifted goods worth twenty dollars or more; 5 percent had committed break-and-enter, and 5 percent had stolen a motor vehicle. This study identified high levels of truancy, cannabis use, and alcohol use as being the most important factors contributing to student involvement in assault, malicious damage, and property crime. Poor parental supervision was also identified as being an important factor contributing to involvement in malicious damage and property crime, but not in assault.[44]

If there is an overlap between crime and substance abuse, and individuals with ADHD are more prone to crime than others, a logical assumption would be that they are also more likely to abuse alcohol and drugs. Statistics abound that this is indeed the case. Studies have found that nearly 40 percent of all cocaine and opiate abusers meet the diagnostic criteria for ADHD.[45] In comparison to other opiate and cocaine abusers, those with a history of ADHD generally began their abuse at an earlier age and exhibited more severe abusing habits. Research also suggests that one-third of adults with ADHD abuse alcohol,[46] and that individuals with ADHD are as much as seven times more likely than others to abuse drugs in adulthood.[47]

Although these statistics should especially concern parents whose children have been diagnosed with ADHD, it should be the aim of *every* parent to protect children from alcohol and drugs. Both are easy to come by, and today's children—ADHD or not—are put under tremendous peer and societal pressure to experiment with them.

Before the 1950s, the social problems of drugs were relatively narrow and confined. Problems existed with heroin in larger cities, marijuana had a small following, some amphetamine abuse existed, but drugs were rarely mentioned as a major social issue.[48] But since then, the situation has changed drastically. According to one source, teenage drug arrests in the United States have risen 1,451 percent since 1965.[49] A 1987 Gallup report indicated that before graduating from high school, a staggering percentage of teenagers were hooked on mind-altering drugs of some type; 85 percent had experimented with alcohol, and 57 percent had tried an illicit drug.[50]

Although the Department of Health and Human Services boasted in 1992 that the nationwide pattern of drug abuse was in decline, revealing an 11 percent dip in illicit drug use by Americans twelve years or older, from 12.8 million in 1991 to 11.4 million in

1992, not everybody was convinced. "The high times may be a-changin', but America's drug scene is as frightening as ever," an article in the *Times* stated:

> Last week the University of Michigan released a survey show-ing a rise in illicit drug use by American college students, with the most significant increase involving hallucinogens like LSD. Meanwhile a canvas of narcotics experts across the country indicated that while drug fashions vary from region to region and class to class, crack use is generally holding steady and heroin and marijuana are on the rise. Junior high and high school students surveyed by the government report a greater availability of most serious drugs. Law officials and treatment specialists on the front lines of the drug war report that the problem transcends both income and racial differ-ences. "When it comes to drugs, there is a complete democ-racy," says Clark Carr. . . .

> Ironically, the heroin surge . . . reflects a new health con-sciousness on the part of drug abusers. Youthful offenders, scared off by the devastation of crack, are dabbling in heroin instead, while chronic crack addicts are changing over to heroin because of its mellower high and cheaper cost. Among both groups, fear of HIV transmission has made snorting, rather than injection, the preferred method of ingestion. "The needle is out, man," says Stephan ("Boobie") Gaston, 40, of East Harlem, a 26-year abuser. "All they're doing is sniffing." Even so, the risks remain high. Heroin-related incidents jumped from 10,300 during a three-month period in 1991 to 13,400 during a comparable period in 1992, according to a Federal Drug Abuse Warning Network survey of hospital emergency rooms. Heroin-treatment admissions have also increased over the past year.[51]

Other sources also seem to confirm that the war against alcohol and drugs are far from over. According to one source, the number of youth arrests for selling illegal drugs, especially marijuana, jumped from 64,740 in 1990 to 147,107 in 1995.[52] The 1997 *Monitoring the Future Study* (MTF) found that 49.6 percent of high school seniors reported having tried marijuana, which continues to be the most frequently used illegal drug, at least once—up from 41.7 percent in 1995. Roughly 40 percent of youngsters ages fifteen to nineteen who enter drug treatment, have marijuana as the primary drug of abuse.

Increasing rates of heroin use among youth are equally frightening. While heroin use among young people remains quite low, use among teens rose significantly in eighth, tenth, and twelfth grades during the 1990s. In each grade, 2.1 percent of students have tried this horrible drug. The average age of initiation for heroin had fallen from 27.3 years in 1988 to 19.3 in 1995. The 1997 MTF survey found that the proportion of students reporting use of powder cocaine in the past year was 2.2, 4.1, and 5 percent in grades eight, ten, and twelve, respectively. "Speedballing," combining heroin with cocaine, is increasingly common. Treatment providers report that 75 percent of clients in heroin treatment report cocaine abuse as well. The 1997 MTF also reported that inhalant use is most common in the eighth grade, where 5.6 percent used it within the past month and 11.8 percent used it in the previous year. Inhalants can also be deadly, even with first-time use, and often represent the initial experience with illicit substances.

Similar concerns are raised by the rate of underage drinking. In 1997, the MTF found that 15 percent of eighth, 25 percent of tenth, and 31 percent of twelfth graders reported binge drinking in the two weeks prior to being interviewed. Between 1996 and 1997, the incidence of binge drinking rose by 15 percent among 12- to 17-year-olds. Heavy drinking has increased by almost 7 percent during the same period.[53]

New research indicates that the younger the age of drinking onset, the greater the chance that an individual at some point in life will develop a "clinically defined alcohol disorder." Young people who began drinking before age fifteen were four times more likely to develop alcohol dependence than those who began drinking at age twenty-one. Here again, underage alcohol use is a risk factor that correlates with higher incidences of drug use among young people.[54]

America, however, is not the only country that needs to worry about its youth. According to the German magazine *Theologisches*, two hundred thousand 14- to 21-year-olds in Germany are alcoholics. Three quarters of the country's teenagers have used hash. The number of people who took hard drugs for the first time tripled from 1983 to 1993. Germany has an estimated twenty thousand skinheads between the ages of eighteen and twenty-five.[55]

The drug-using habits of British schoolchildren also give much cause for concern. Professor Martin Plant, head of the Alcohol and Health Research Group in Edinburgh, recently admitted that "the UK is the drugs capital of Europe."[56]

Probably few countries have seen such an explosion in drug abuse as South Africa, where the situation has reached crisis point in only a few years. In 1991, there was a minuscule number of cases involving cocaine. In 1992, the total value of confiscated cocaine was nearly two million rands (South African currency). In 1994, it was 12.5 million. In the same two year period the total value of confiscated cannabis increased with 48 percent, mandrax with 27 percent, heroin with 1,823 percent and LSD with 352 percent.[57]

In 1996, drugs counselor Gail Hickman stated that

> by the time South African students have reached Grade 12, about 85 percent have had some interaction with drugs. This doesn't mean all 85 percent are drug users but that some of them are taking drugs, some have a family member who does drugs and the rest have had some connection or other with drugs—for instance, attended a party where there was a lot of drugging taking place. Of the 85 percent, 60 percent will become fairly regular to regular users. Of them, as many as 30 percent will eventually become addicts.

These children, desperate for cocaine, heroin, LSD, and Ecstasy—the drug that has become synonymous with the latest youth phenomenon, the rave scene—will do literally anything to obtain money for the drugs, says Hickman:

> They won't hesitate to steal it from their parents, or goods from the home or store in order to get it. If you're a girl you don't need to steal money, you simply use your young, supple body. These poor misguided girls don't actually get paid for the sex, they simply exchange sexual favors for drugs. So they'll have sex with any man who's prepared to share his drugs with them—which is often the dealer. Such girls are known as drug sluts in the underworld and are usually between 13- and 18-years old. They're no better than prostitutes—though they don't think they're in the same category because many of them come from good families and plush areas.

A lot of sex takes place in the clubs—in storerooms, back offices, alleys and even in some corners in the clubs. "The girls aren't choosy who they sleep with," says Hickman. "Anything goes as long as the reward is an E-tablet, cocaine, or whatever. Condoms aren't a major consideration for them, either. There's so much unsafe sex taking place among teenagers that it's frightening. Most kids have heard of AIDS but not of other sexually transmitted diseases. Mention syphilis or gonorrhea to them and they look puzzled. Those diseases don't seem to scare anyone any more."[58]

In January 1999, a newspaper revealed that the number of South African youths admitted for treatment on account of drug abuse has increased by 50 percent since 1996. The newspaper also revealed that a survey conducted in 1996 at two hundred schools found that one in every three children was involved in drugs. When the survey was repeated at these schools in 1998, the number was two in three. Drugs in South Africa are no longer a problem associated with high school. Users are often as young as ten.[59]

The Epidemic of Teenage Promiscuity

Unwed motherhood is increasing rapidly in virtually every part of the developed world. The percentage of non-marital births in the United States approximately doubled from 14.2 percent in 1975[60] to almost 30 percent in 1991.[61] The rate of increase was about as steep—and, in some cases, steeper—in Canada and many European countries. In six northern European countries, the percentage of non-marital births in 1990 averaged 33.3 percent.[62]

At present, the United States leads the developed world in the percentage of single-parent households with dependent children, but other developed countries—notably Sweden, Australia, and the United Kingdom—are experiencing similar problems. The United States also leads the developed world in divorce rates, but the rate of increase is higher in other countries. The divorce rates more than doubled between 1970 and 1990 in Canada, England and Wales, France, Greece, the Netherlands, and the former West Germany.[63]

Contrary to the 1960s when it was 9 percent, 27 percent of the families in America are now headed by a single parent, usually the mother.[64] Most of the children in these families were born to teenagers.

Between 1960 and 1991, unwed pregnancies have increased 310 percent among 15- to 19-year-olds.[65] At present, one in ten American teenage females—12 percent of all female teenagers and 21 percent of those who have had sexual intercourse—become pregnant annually,[66] which adds up to more than three thousand a day.[67] Of these more than three thousand pregnancies per day, approximately 46 percent result in live births, 41 percent are aborted[68] (an increase of 67 percent since 1973)[69] and the remainder end in miscarriage or stillbirth. One of four teenage mothers will have a second child within one year of her first child's birth.[70]

The economic and social cost of this epidemic is staggering. Most teen mothers are single and receive no support from the father. Eight of ten teenage mothers do not finish high school. According to the Center for Disease Control, 85 percent of all children exhibiting behavioral disorders come from fatherless homes. Other statistical findings indicate that children from fatherless homes are thirty-two times more likely to run away; nine times more likely to drop out of high school; fourteen times more likely to commit rape; ten times more likely to be substance abusers; and twenty times more likely to end up in prison.[71]

Besides breeding another lost generation of children, the growing sexual promiscuity among the youth carries the potential of tremendous health problems. Sexually transmitted diseases are now infecting three million American teenagers annually.[72]

The Horror Statistics of Suicide

The suicide rate among American youth, especially those 15- to 24-years-old, has increased dramatically during the past three decades. From 1957 to 1987 the suicide rate for 15- to 24-year-olds increased from 4 to 12.9 per 100,000. During the same period, the suicide rate for the general population rose from 9.8 to 12.7 per one hundred thousand.[73] Today, suicide is the second leading cause of death for 15- to 24-year-olds.[74] The leading cause of death in this age group is automobile accidents, of which the majority is related to alcohol abuse. The suicide rate for American 10- to 14-year-olds increased by 190 percent between 1963 and 1995, from 0.6 to 1.74 per one hundred thousand.[75]

In Britain, suicide has overtaken automobile accidents as the main cause of death among young men in some parts of Britain, and is now one of the country's biggest public health problems. Suicide rates among young men aged 15 to 24 rose 80 percent between 1980 and 1992. Although they have since declined slightly, in 1996 suicide was still 55 percent above its level in 1983, claiming 1,000 lives a year in this age group. Three quarters of all suicide cases are men. Among those aged 15 to 24 who kill themselves, 80 percent are men. Even though a poll found that most men would seek help from their doctors, rather than from family, friends, or helplines if they were thinking of suicide, more than four million calls a year are made to the Samaritans, one of the British helplines.[76]

A United Nations report, *The Progress of Nations,* recently ranked New Zealand as having one of the highest teenage suicide rates among industrialized countries.[77] Suicide in the fifteen to nineteen age group has increased over the last twenty years, from 5.8 per one hundred thousand in 1970 to 15.7 in 1991. In 1991, the suicide rate for the twenty to twenty-four age group was 31.3 per one hundred thousand, with the increase much higher among males than females.[78] Other Western countries with high suicide rates—twenty per one hundred thousand inhabitants or higher—include Finland, Austria, Sweden, Denmark, and Germany. In Canada, the suicide rate is roughly comparable to that of the United States.[79]

Although official suicide rates are evidence of the magnitude of the problem, they do not give a complete picture of this phenomenon. For every teenager who is recorded as having completed suicide, many more have attempted it. A 1990 Gallup survey found that 15 percent of American teenagers had considered suicide at some time, and that 6 percent had actually attempted it.[80] And while young males tend to successfully kill themselves, significantly more women attempt suicide.[81] Also, even though statistics show increasing rates of suicide among young people, they do not show that suicides are probably underreported because coroners often have difficulty deciding whether a death was due to suicide and may not report it as such.[82]

The Canterbury Suicide Project investigated individual histories of suicides and attempted suicides in New Zealand. Preliminary findings identified high rates of *depression, antisocial behavior, and alcohol and drug problems.*[83] Although it is by no means encouraging, one cannot ignore the fact that these risk factors are all predominant of ADHD.

The Erosion of Education

At the beginning of the twentieth century, academic achievement in the United States and elsewhere was excellent. Compulsory schooling, and the continuous rise of educational standards were the Western world's admissions to literacy and intelligence and for the first five decades of the twentieth century a source of pride. Yet, as Lionni and Klass point out, "Somewhere along the line our schools had lost the ability to routinely educate children and produce uniformly good results."[84]

The erosion of America's educational performance, which by now has reached crisis point at all levels, is summarized in a 1976 *Los Angeles* article:

After edging upward for apparently more than a century, the reading, writing, and mathematical skills of American students from elementary school through college are now in a prolonged and broad scale decline unequaled in history. The downward spiral, which affects many other subject areas as well, began abruptly in the mid-1960s and shows no signs of bottoming out.[85]

In 1910, only 2.2 percent of American children between the ages of ten and fourteen could neither read nor write. It is important to note that the illiteracy of 1910 reflected, for the most part, children who never had the advantage of schooling. The illiterates of today, however, are not people who never went to school. They are predominantly individuals who have spent eight to twelve years in public schools.[86]

According to the National Adult Literacy Survey, 42 million adult Americans cannot read; fifty million can recognize so few printed words they are limited to a fourth or fifth grade reading level; one out of every four teenagers drops out of high school, and, of those who graduate, one out of every four has the equivalent or less of an eighth grade education.[87] Writing in the monthly *Commentary*, Chester E. Finn, Jr., a professor at Vanderbilt University, cites the dismal findings of the National Assessment of Educational Progress. "Just 5 percent of 17-year-old high school students can read well enough to understand and use information found in technical materials, literary essays, and historical documents." Imagine how hopeless it is to get the other 95 percent to read Plato or Shakespeare or the Bible. "Barely 6 percent of them," Finn continues, "can solve multistep math problems and use basic algebra." We're not talking difficult math here but rather something as elementary as calculating simple interest on a loan.[88]

While illiteracy has been, and is still growing, on the one hand, the standards of education have been declining—tragically and steadily—on the other. Reading levels of young Americans fell so low in the 1970s that the Army was forced to rewrite its operating manuals in comic fashion.[89] Much reading material, previously used for years in American schools, became incomprehensible to present-day students and had to be simplified. For example, when a well-known history book was revised with an eye toward the high school market, words like "spectacle" and "admired" were removed. Apparently they were too difficult.[90]

Universities were also affected. As Sydney J. Harris put it, "For the first hundred years of its existence, a college like Harvard would not graduate a student without a knowledge of Hebrew. Now the point is approaching when one can be graduated without a knowledge of English."[91]

There is a growing body of evidence that suggests that many of the American public school teachers are themselves woefully undereducated. In 1983, for example, schoolteachers in Houston, Texas, were required to take a competency test. More than 60 percent of the teachers failed the reading part of the test; 46 percent failed the math section, while 26 percent failed the writing section. As if this weren't bad enough, 763 of the more than 3,000 teachers taking the test cheated.[92]

Peter S. Prescott, writing in *Newsweek*, said, "The fashion of our present time is to know less and less about more and more." Lewis Mumford, after more than a half-century of reflection, concluded, "I have a book on my shelves by a man who says that the Dark Age is coming. I think the Dark Age is already here, only we don't know it."[93]

The "Dark Age," however, is not confined to America. In Australia, there is widespread agreement that something is drastically wrong with Australian schools and universities.[94] The percentage of schoolchildren that could read and write increased from 59.1 percent in 1871, to 79.8 percent in 1901, and 90.2 percent in 1911.[95] But somewhere along the line something must have happened. A survey in the 1970s of several high schools in the Sydney metropolitan area, has shown that 22.8 percent of the first form (seventh grade) students interviewed had reading ages of nine or younger. The Bonorian High School advisory center in Victoria surveyed more than twenty-six hundred students in first and second forms in twelve eastern suburb high schools. The results showed that 45.7 percent of those tested needed remedial specialist training if they were to profit from high school work, and 25 percent were found to read so badly as to be classified illiterate. Both surveys excluded children with acknowledged lower intelligence and migrant background.[96] And in 1990, a survey of Australian adult literacy, reported in *The Australian*, found that "70 percent of a representative group of adults could not deal with concepts or arguments at the level of a standard newspaper editorial."[97]

Meanwhile, in Britain, more than two million people are said to be completely illiterate, according to a UNESCO report. More than a third of the 11-year-old children arriving at many secondary schools in Britain's inner cities are such poor readers that they cannot properly understand their textbooks.[98]

Yearly, the lives of millions of Western children are wasted. But even more so is the life of the child with ADHD, as this "disorder" has devastating effects on intellectual functioning. As it has already been stated, 80 percent of children with ADHD have problems with reading, spelling, and writing. Research also demonstrates that ADHD has a negative impact on intelligence (an average of seven to ten points below normal), on academic achievement skills (an average of ten to fifteen points below normal), and on academic progress (25 to 50 percent are retained in grade, 36 percent fail to graduate high school, and only 5 percent complete a college education).[99]

We simply cannot allow the plight of the ADHD child to continue any longer. We *have* to make an end to this foolishness. We have no other choice, but to put the creators of ADHD—and of youth violence, the drug culture, teenage promiscuity, the wave of teen suicides, and illiteracy—on trial.

Notes

1. Adams, J. E., *Competent to Counsel* (Philipsburg, New Jersey: Presbyterian and Reformed Publishing Company, 1970), 1.

2. "Religion under attack," *Psychiatry Destroying Religion* (Los Angeles: CCHR, 1997), 4-7.

3. Ibid.

4. Sunter, C., *The High Road: Where Are We Now?* (Cape Town: Tafelberg, Human & Rousseau (Pty.) Ltd., 1996), 71.

5. "Religion under attack," *Psychiatry Destroying Religion*.

6. Sunter, *The High Road*, 71-72.

7. "Religion under attack," *Psychiatry Destroying Religion*.

8. Ibid.

9. Sunter, *The High Road*, 71.

10. "Religion under attack," *Psychiatry Destroying Religion*.

11. Sunter, *The High Road*, 72.

12. Page, C., "Law finding better ways to deal with juvenile crime," *The Dallas Morning News*, 18 August 1996, 5J.

13. "The school of death," *The Star*, 22 April 1999, 1.

14. Ourlian, R., et al., "Youth: Recent spate stands out all the more as the overall teen crime rate drops," *Los Angeles Times*, 14 March 1999.

15. Edwards, R., "The search for a proper punishment. Psychologists add fuel to the debate over whether young offenders should be tried as adults," website of the American Psychological Association.

16. Newton, M., *Mass Murder. An Annotated Biography* (New York: Garland, 1985).

17. Wilkerson, I., "Two boys, a debt, a gun, a victim. The face of violence," *New York Times*, 16 May 1994.

18. Bennett, W., *Index of Leading Cultural Indicators*, cited in "100 Harshest facts about our future," 1997; *Sourcebook of Criminal Justice Statistics: 1993* (Bureau of Justice Statistics: U.S. Department of Justice), 327, cited in B. Wiseman, *Psychiatry: The Ultimate Betrayal* (Los Angeles: Freedom Publishing, 1995), 227.

19. Edwards, "The search for a proper punishment."

20. Coleman, J. C., Butcher, J. N., & Carson, R. C., *Abnormal Psychology and Modern Life* (7th ed.), (Glenview, Illinois: Scott, Foresman and Company, 1984), 550.

21. Manning, S., "A national emergency," *Scholastic Update*, 5 April 1991, 2.

22. "Uniform Crime Reports," United States Department of Justice, 1992.

23. Lacayo, R., "When kids go bad," *Time*, 19 September 1994, 60-63.

24. "Juristat," Service Bulletin for the Canadian Center for Justice Statistics, October 1990, cited in "Illiteracy and crime: An international problem," *Psychiatry: Education's Ruin* (Los Angeles: CCHR, 1995), 20-21.

25. "Education: Violence," *Canada and the World Backgrounder*, 1 December 1998.

26. Carey, E., "Crimes by girls on rise: Study," *The Toronto Star*, 16 December 1998.

27. "Education: Violence," *Canada and the World Backgrounder*.

28. Toynbee, P., "Crime is up! Hit the moral panic button," *Independent*, 25 September 1996, 15.

29. Britain violent crime statistics, 1960-1993, cited in "Illiteracy and crime: An international problem," *Psychiatry: Education's Ruin.*

30. Toynbee, "Crime is up! Hit the moral panic button."

31. Fowler, R., "Girls get violent," *Independent*, 2 May 1996, 15.

32. Ibid.

33. "France: The kids' revolt," *The Economist*, vol. 346, 1998.

34. Australian crime statistics, Number of offences reported to police for "serious assault," 1973-74 to 1991-92.

35. New Zealand violent crime statistics, 1960-1990, cited in "Illiteracy and crime: An international problem," *Psychiatry: Education's Ruin.*

36. "Crime: UK tops EC crime rate," *Europe 2000-Human Resources.*

37. "The crime decline: Yes and no," *The World & I*, vol. 12, 10 January 1997, 20.

38. "Number of offences reported per 100,000 population for selected countries, 1972-1985," *The Size of the Crime Problem in Australia.*

39. "Our children cast adrift," *Psychiatry: Betraying and Drugging Children* (Los Angeles: CCHR, 1998), 24-29.

40. "Germany reports sharp rise in juvenile delinquencies," *Xinhua News*, 29 May 1998.

41. Mannuzza, S., Klein, R., Bonagura, N., Malloy, P., Giampino, T. L., & Addalli, K. A., "Hyperactive boys almost grown up: IV. Criminality and its relationship to psychiatric status," *Archives of General Psychiatry*, vol. 46, 1989, 1073-1079, cited in S. Goldstein, "Attention-deficit/ hyperactivity disorder: Implications for the criminal justice system," *The FBI Law Enforcement Bulletin*, vol. 66, 1997, 11-16.

42. Ibid.

43. "Drug-Facts," *Executive News Service*, 1989, cited in Wiseman, *Psychiatry: The Ultimate Betrayal*, 247.

44. "Participation rates and risk factors," *Juveniles in Crime*, Part 1, December 1998.

45. Cocores, J. A., Davies, R. K., Mueller, P. S., & Gold, M. S., "Cocaine abuse and adult Attention-Deficit Disorder," *Journal of Clinical Psychiatry*, vol. 48, 376-377, cited in Goldstein, "Attention-deficit/hyperactivity disorder."

46. Goldstein, "Attention-deficit/hyperactivity disorder."

47. Mannuzza, et al., "Hyperactive boys almost grown up: IV. Criminality and its relationship to psychiatric status," cited in Goldstein, "Attention-deficit/hyperactivity disorder."

48. "LSD: Psychiatry controlling culture," *Psychiatry Manipulating Creativity* (Los Angeles: CCHR, 1997), 22-25.

49. "Psychiatry destroys futures," *Psychiatry Manipulating Creativity* (Los Angeles: CCHR, 1997), 46-49.

50. "Alcohol use and abuse in America," *Gallup Report,* No. 265, 1987, 3.

51. Smolowe, J., "Drugs: Choose your poison," *Time,* 26 July 1993, 56.

52. "Psychiatry destroys futures," *Psychiatry Manipulating Creativity.*

53. McCaffrey, B. R., "Drug abuse among children," *Congressional Testimony,* 17 June 1998.

54. Ibid.

55. Meves, C., *Theologisches,* vol. 24(6), 267-268, cited in "Psychiatry eradicates morals," *Psychiatry Destroying Religion* (Los Angeles: CCHR, 1997), 54-61.

56. Burrell, I., "Britain is the drugs capital of Europe," *Independent,* 3 November 1997, 1.

57. *Beeld,* 25 January 1997.

58. Zonga, A., "Partying to death," *Personality,* 11 October 1996, 26-29.

59. Badenhorst, E., "Dwelms vat skole oor," *Rapport,* 24 January 1999, 1.

60. "Changes in family life not unique to U.S.," *Contemporary Women's Issues Database,* 1 September 1995.

61. National Center for Health Statistics, 1993.

62. "Changes in family life not unique to U.S.," *Contemporary Women's Issues.*

63. Ibid.

64. *Marriage in America: A Report to the Nation* (New York: Institute for American Values, 1995).

65. "Psychiatry eradicates morals," *Psychiatry Destroying Religion.*

66. Henshaw, "U.S. teenage pregnancy statistics," *AGI,* New York, 1993.

67. Stephens, G., "Youth at risk: Saving the world's most precious resource," *The Futurist,* vol. 31, 1997.

68. Baber, K. M., "Adolescent pregnancy and parenthood," in S. J. Price, P. C. McKenry & S. Gavazzi (eds.), *Vision 2010: Families and Adolescents* (Minnesota: National Council on Family Relations, 1994).

69. Crouse, G. L., Office of Planning and Evaluation, U.S. Department of Health & Human Services, cited in J. Dobson, *The New Dare to Discipline* (Wheaton, Illinois: Tyndale House Publishers, Inc., 1992), 212.

70. Stephens, "Youth at risk."

71. Ibid.

72. "Heterosexual HIV transmission up in the United States," *American Medical News,* 3 February 1992, cited in Dobson, *The New Dare to Discipline,* 209.

73. Zhang, J., & Jin, S., "Determinants of suicide ideation: a comparison of Chinese and American college students," *Adolescence,* vol. 31, 1 June 1996, 451-467.

74. "Our children cast adrift," *Psychiatry: Betraying and Drugging Children.*

75. Ibid.

76. Laurance, J., "Suicide toll higher than road deaths," *Independent,* 24 February 1999.

77. *The Progress of Nations* (New York: UNICEF, 1994).

78. Aldrigde, V., "The horror statistics of suicide," *The Dominion,* July 1994, 11.

79. Coleman, et al., *Abnormal Psychology and Modern Life,* 328-329.

80. Walsh, D., *Selling Out America's Children: How America Puts Profits before Values—And What Parents Can Do* (Minneapolis: Fairview Press, 1995).

81. Tan, M., *An Analysis of Suicide Attempts in 1980-1988* (Massey University: Thesis, 1991).

82. "Adolescents at risk: causes of youth suicide in New Zealand," *Adolescence,* 22 December 1997.

83. Ibid.

84. Lionni, P., & Klass, L. J., *The Leipzig Connection: The Systematic Destruction of American Education* (Portland, Oregon: Heron Books, 1980).

85. McCurdy, J., & Speich, D., "Student skills decline unequalled in history," *Los Angeles Times*, 15 August 1976, cited in "Education and social ruin," *Education: Psychiatry's Ruin* (Los Angeles: CCHR, 1995), 2-3.

86. Nash, R. H., "The three kinds of illiteracy," 1999, www. christiananswers.net/summit/nashtki.html.

87. Sweet, R. W., "Illiteracy: An incurable disease or education malpractice," The National Right to Read Foundation, 1996, www.nrrf.org/essays.html.

88. Chester, F., "A nation still at risk," *Commentary*, no. 87, May 1989, cited in Nash, "The three kinds of illiteracy."

89. Honig, B., *Last Chance for Our Children* (New York: Addison-Wesley Publishing, Inc., 1987), ix.

90. O'Brien, S., "The reshaping of history: Marketers v. authors," *Cirriculum Review*, September 1988, 11, cited in T. Sowell, *Inside American Education* (Englewood Cliffs: Julian Messner, 1993), 7.

91. Lean, A. E., & Eaton, W. E., *Education or Catastrophe?* (Wolfeboro: Longwood Academic, 1990), 28.

92. Nash, "The three kinds of illiteracy."

93. Lean & Eaton, *Education or Catastrophe?* 31.

94. Frodsham, J. D., "Introduction," in J. D. Frodsham (ed.), *Education for What?* (Canberra: Academy Press, 1990), 1-10.

95. *Commonwealth Year Book 1924*, 477-478, cited in J. Lawry, Cleverly & Lawry (eds.), *Australian Education in the 20th Century* (Longman, 1972), 1-2.

96. Wallis, J. M., *The Disaster Road* (Bullsbrook: Veritas Publishing Company Pty. Ltd., 1986), 92.

97. Frodsham, "Introduction."

98. "Illiteracy and crime: An international problem," *Education: Psychiatry's Ruin*.

99. Barkley, R. A., "ADHD, Ritalin, and conspiracies: Talking back to Peter Breggin," Russell Barkley Book Review, CH.A.A.D., www.catalog.com/chadd/news/Russ-review.htm.

7.

The Soulless
Roots of Psychology and Psychiatry

Scientists and physicians are the miracle workers of our century, having provided everything from electric light against the darkness to a vaccine against polio. Their technical inventiveness seems capable of mastering the physical universe. In America, we tend to hold them in high regard as impartial, humane, and above all, objective. "Doctor-recommended" highlights many advertisements. We expect physicians and scientists to deal with facts—precise bits of physical evidence that are indisputable.[1]

Against this background of expectations and beliefs, scientists and doctors are attempting to address violence as a disease. Federal agencies, foundations, and private industry are pouring hundreds of millions of dollars into the search for a biological basis for violent crime and antisocial behavior. Once it is found, drug treatments can be developed and administered to those who are biologically or genetically disposed to violence.[2]

Thousands of children, in conflict with their parents, schools, and society are routinely subjected to biochemical research involving spinal taps, brain scans, and other invasive procedures. Frequently they are subjected to toxic or experimental medications for the control of their behavior.[3]

Three studies on children recently came to light in which a hundred children from seven- to ten-years-old, mostly black or Hispanic, were brought into clinics and injected with the now-banned diet drug, fenfluramine. The object was to provoke the production of a brain chemical that scientists believe is linked to aggression and violence. It is this kind of research that has urged Vera Sharav, director of Citizens for Responsible Care in Psychiatry and Research—a New York advocacy group, who has brought many such imprudent studies to light—to state that psychiatric research is "out of control."[4]

If one considers the violence surrounding us, as well as the increasing number of children who are in conflict with authority, it becomes evident that medical science is still far removed from any breakthrough regarding a biological basis for violence and antisocial behavior, not to mention an effective preventive drug. When will it ever dawn on them that they have not found a biological basis, and probably never will, simply because such a basis most likely does not exist? Isn't it time for them to look for *another* explanation for these problems? If a theory is in no way substantiated or verified by practical results, wouldn't a logical step be to *discard* it, and *replace it with a new one?* An example should make this clear.

Suppose that you are driving from one place to another, and your car suddenly stalls and stops. Suppose further that you conclude that you have run out of fuel. Such a conclusion would be your theory, i.e., your tentative explanation for the unexpected stopping of the car. Just having a theory, however, does not solve the problem yet. You now have to act according to this theory, to discover whether the theory will be of any help in solving the problem. The easiest thing to do would be to thumb a ride to the nearest filling station, to come back with a can of fuel to pour into the tank. If the car starts, then your theory has at least been proven useful in your attempt to solve the problem. (Note that we use the words "proven *useful*" because, even if the car starts after you have poured fuel into the tank, it does not necessarily prove the *correctness* of your theory beyond any doubt. The trouble could also have been caused, for example, by an overheated engine, which had cooled down in the meantime.)

The important point that we wish to illustrate by means of this example is that if the car does *not* start when you come back with the can of fuel, it would certainly serve no purpose to return for another can of fuel. That, however, is exactly what is being done to children. The promoters of the biological idea obstinately stick to their pet theory, although its uselessness has been proven over and over—and over. We cannot accept that stupidity alone can be the only reason for this stubborn attitude. There has to be some other explanation. One possibility is that, although the biological model has proven to be quite useless to help the children in any way, it has proven to be very useful indeed as a money-making idea. There may, of course, also be some other hidden agenda that is served by ruining all children, thereby gradually but inexorably bringing the whole of Western civilization to its knees.

For parents, however, who wish to help their children, the only solution would be to try a *different* possibility. To a great extent this idea—to replace a theory with a new one if it does not produce practical results—is incompatible with the modern view on science, in which the scientific *method* is considered to be of far greater importance than the *results*.[5]

In more than half a century, the theory that a behavior or social problem—whether ADHD, ODD, CD or any other related problem—is biologically or neurologically based, could not produce any tangible results in practice. Instead of replacing this theory with another theory, it seems that the only concern is that the research methods must be valid. Apart from the fact that they are making a lot of money out of the children's plight, it seems that the attitude of the scientists is that the method is of greater importance than the well-being of the child. Only the methodology counts, even if the ideas underlying these methods are pure nonsense, and even if these methods lead to nothing at all.

When dealing with the child who experiences behavioral difficulties, it is the end result that really matters, whether the child is enabled to improve his behavior. No matter how much time and effort one expends in checking the scientific rigor of all methods and procedures that are employed in an effort to help the child; if, in the end, he is not helped to lead a productive life, it was all a useless waste of time as far as the child is concerned.

Before it becomes possible to formulate another *accountable* theory, which aims at explaining these problems, however, it will be necessary to study the *view of man.* Man's view of himself determines the direction in which he moves. When the Israelites, for example, viewed themselves as God's chosen people, they obeyed God's laws. When they lost this view, they adopted pagan habits.

Members of the Psychological Guild on the Stand

Psychology and psychiatry have become an integral part of Western society. "From entertainment to news, television is enthralled, awestruck and dazzled by the mysteries of virtually anything that smacks of psychiatry and psychology," wrote Dr. Thomas Szasz.[6] The schools are flooded by practitioners, in courtrooms they argue for the acquittal of criminal defendants, and theological colleges and seminaries enthusiastically encourage Christians to submit to the insights, methods and findings of psychology. In short, the world is in love with psychology and its cousin, psychiatry.

However, not everybody is convinced of the virtues of psychological and psychiatric ideas. There are certainly those who would designate them as devils in sheep's clothing.

Michael Skube wrote:

> Every profession, I suppose, has its quacks and charlatans, but I sometimes wonder if we are better off for having psychologists. I don't think we are. I have known psychologists who were perfectly decent people, and intelligent enough to be interesting. But individual practitioners are one thing and the profession another. Psychology is a pseudoscience that cannot point to a body of real knowledge, and yet people take it in, convinced that their children have learning disabilities when they don't, recalling traumatic events that never happened until their therapist said they did.[7]

As Michael Skube is only a journalist, his criticism could perhaps be shrugged off. Some would be inclined to say that he is merely showing his ignorance. It is interesting to note, however, that some of the most outspoken critics against psychology and psychiatry are not journalists, but *psychologists* and *psychiatrists*, many of whom have practiced for a great number of years.

In *The Death of Psychiatry* (1974), psychiatrist Torrey acknowledged, for example, that psychological labels "are impressive and convey to the uninitiated that we know what we are talking about. Unfortunately, this is not the case."[8]

In *Against Therapy* (1988), Jeffrey Masson, a former psychoanalyst, reported that psychoanalytical training does not prepare a person to be a better counselor. He testified that after five years of intensive analysis on himself and his patients he did not understand "emotional problems of living" better than people with no training. Masson's thesis is that all therapy is unneeded and long years of intensive psychological study are a waste of time: "I spent eight years in my psychoanalytical training. In retrospect, I feel I could have learned the basic ideas in about eight hours of concentrated reading."[9]

In 1988, Gary Collins' *Can You Trust Psychology?* was published. He starts his first chapter with the following statement:

Bernie Zilbergeld doesn't trust psychology. Despite his Ph.D. from Berkeley, his twelve years' experience as a practicing therapist, and his acclaim as a psychological researcher and author, Dr. Zilbergeld has written a whole book to criticize his own profession. Many psychological conclusions are really myths, he writes. Professional therapy is "overpromoted, overused and overvalued." These criticisms could be dismissed had they come instead from a journalist or theologian writing as an outsider. But they come instead from a member of the psychological guild who has gone through all the prescribed training in clinical psychology, has been in therapy himself, has taken the time to interview 140 former patients, and has met for lengthy discussions with a cross-range of fourteen professional colleagues.[10]

In 1993, in an interview, Dr. Thomas Szasz stated, "Psychiatry is probably the single most destructive force that has affected the American society within the last fifty years." Dr. Szasz, an outspoken critic of his profession, was not limiting this comment to the confines of the psychiatric hospital and couch. He was talking about the decline of our entire social structure. "Psychiatry is a part of the general liberal ethos," he added. "You know, everybody is a victim, everybody has special rights, no responsibilities. This psychiatric view has so completely infiltrated American thinking, people don't even think of it as psychiatry."[11]

More recently, in *House of Cards: Psychology and Psychotherapy Built on Myth,* Robyn M. Dawes, a psychologist, deplored the errors of psychologists' ways. His targets included:

> . . . psychological "experts" (there is so little known that there is nothing to be expert about), clinicians who boast about their "experience" (research shows experienced people do no better than amateurs at making diagnoses and providing therapy), psychological licensure (licensed people are not more competent or ethical than others), psychological testimony in courts of law (almost always based on impressions, perceptions, intuitions, personal experience, and other invalid sources of knowledge), . . . self-esteem ("the holy grail" of pop psychology is a "mirage"), American education (teachers are so busy working on kids' self-esteem that there's no time left to teach anything) and psychological professionalism in general (faddish, unscientific, contemptuous, greedy, and self-serving).[12]

The question to be answered is why these scholars would criticize their own professions? What is wrong with psychiatry? And what could be wrong with psychology?

What is wrong—in short—is that *psychology*, which originated as a religious study—psychology means the "study of the soul"—has become a "science without a soul."[13] And so has *psychiatry*, a term first coined in 1808 by Johann Christian Bell, meaning "doctoring of the soul." Psychology lost its "soul" in 1879, when a "new" or "modern" psychology originated at Leipzig University, Germany, in the person of Wilhelm Wundt. Wundt conducted research in a field he founded and called "experimental psychology." Leipzig soon became the Mecca of students who wished to study the "new" psychology:

> For the psychology of Leipzig was, in the eighties and nineties, the newest thing under the sun. It was the psychology for bold young radicals who believed that the ways of the mind could be measured and treated experimentally—and who possibly thought of themselves, in their private reflections, as pioneers on the newest frontier of science, pushing its method into reaches of experience that it had never before invaded. At any rate, they threw themselves into their tasks with industry and zest.[14]

Many of Wundt's American students returned to start departments of psychology in major American universities. This was not difficult, since the distinction of having studied under Wundt in Germany carried with it a prestige that made them much sought-after. Wundt's disciples taught hundreds of students on their own, establishing Ph.D. programs that were, in turn, replicated all over the United States.[15]

To appreciate the current influence of "modern" psychological thinking and practice over the people, families and schools of the world, and to understand how it created ADHD, youth violence, the drug culture, teenage promiscuity, the wave of teenage suicides, and illiteracy, it is necessary to first study its roots. As previously stated, the present can only be fully understood if one examines its roots in the past.

The Roots of "Modern" Psychology and Psychiatry

The first root of modern psychology—and of psychiatry—can be found in another pseudoscience, *phrenology*.

In the late eighteenth century, an Austrian physicist, Franz Joseph Gall, introduced an exciting new science, explaining the human mind and behavior. According to Gall, the shape of an individual's skull could identify his moral and intellectual qualities. Named *phrenology* by his pupil Spurzheim, it was believed that a skilled phrenologist could appraise the moral and intellectual qualities of an individual by inspection of the skull, palpating its surface for characteristic bumps or protuberances and depressions.

By the mid-nineteenth century, every major American city had a Phrenology Institute. Illnesses were diagnosed by head-feelers, and companies had potential employees "read" by a phrenologist before they were taken on. Feeling each others' bumps was a jolly way to spend a rainy evening, and even Queen Victoria had her children's heads "read."[16] Even though its fundamental basis was discredited long before, phrenology continued to be practiced until the 1930s, by which time Americans could even have their head bumps read by an automatic electrical phrenology machine which printed out a report on ticker-tape.[17]

In a tongue-in-the-cheek manner, Kevin Kelm recently introduced a technique of "Phrenotherapy." The idea of this "bold new discipline," as its inventor describes it, is to improve people's personalities by rearranging their headbumps—with a mallet![18]

Although it is viewed as a pseudoscience today, phrenology had a large following in the nineteenth century. People accepted this scientific pretender because it seemed to explain why man acts the way he does without making him morally responsible.[19] Even though we make fun of this practice today, it was the forerunner of another group of practices: psychoanalysis, psychiatry, and psychology. While phrenology was losing face, brain analysis of a different kind was catching on in universities. New, powerful microscopes gave rise to a fashion for anatomical dissection. Scientists—including the young Freud—were scrutinizing brain tissue for clues to the physical roots of behavior.[20] "Using more sophisticated techniques to convince the public that they are scientific," says Bulkley, "these new theories [referring to psychological theories] have pulled off a massive deception in our day."[21]

The second root of psychology and its cousin can be found in the advent of the philosophy of materialism—a philosophy that molded a new view of man. One historian, J. R. Kantor, tells us,

> No factor in the evolution of scientific psychology stands
> out more prominently than the doctrines of French Materi-
> alism in the eighteenth century and German Materialism in
> the nineteenth century. . . . Materialism is essentially a non-
> scientific movement, a phenomenon of social transformation
> and change. In the religious domain a materialist is simply
> an atheist.[22]

Materialism is the idea that nothing exists but matter, the physical. There is no God, no soul, and no validity to religion and its
accompanying moral stance.[23] In 1882, Nietzsche made his notori-
ous deliverance, which summarizes the materialistic view of the
Divinity: "God is dead. God remains dead. And we have killed
him." A few years before Nietzsche's publication, in 1859, a book
entitled *The Origin of Species* hit the bookstores. So many people had
with so much expectation looked forward to this book, that its first
edition was sold out on the first day of publication. In this book,
Charles Darwin, the author, claimed that man has evolved from the
animal, and that there were thus only quantitative and no qualitative
differences between man and animals.

The Darwinian theory of evolution has always had a great
power of attraction and conviction for many people, especially physical
scientists, because the final victory of science would be definitive
proof of the origin of man. Before the time of Darwin, people had
to be satisfied with the story of creation as the only explanation for
the origin of man. Anybody who was unwilling to accept the story
of creation—unless he was willing to accept one of the mythologies,
such as the Greek—had to be satisfied with "I don't know." Since
Darwin, the controversy surrounding the origin of man has to a
great extent been limited to evolution and the story of creation.

Evolution is frequently presented as "a scientifically proven fact."
For anybody who accepts this theory as a fact, it would be advisable
to read Richard Milton's book, *The Facts of Life: Shattering the Myths
of Darwinism* (1993). He points out, for example, that the currently
accepted methods of dating are "seriously flawed," and "are supported by Darwinists only because they provide the billions of years
required by Darwinist theories."[24] At the end of his book, Milton
admits that he himself does not know how man originated, but that
the theory of evolution, just as the story of creation, is a matter of
faith or belief. At best, the theory of evolution is thus an ideology
and not a science.

In his book *Secrets of the Lost Races,* Rene Noorbergen points out that a steadily increasing number of historical and archaeological discoveries around the globe suggest that there may have been a period in human history when there was a civilization that was comparable or possibly more advanced than our present society. Of course, the idea of regression, indicated by these "out-of-place" artifacts, does not fit the theory of evolution. Instead of taking another look at their theory, however, evolutionists seem to have no compunction about distorting the facts to fit their theory. According to some evolutionists, these artifacts were left behind by beings from other galaxies who supposedly visited this planet more than ten thousand years ago.[25]

Noorbergen's book makes for interesting reading. His explanation for these "out-of-place" artifacts is that they are the leftovers of a worldwide catastrophe in the distant past—in all probability a flood as described in Genesis—which destroyed a civilization comparable to ours.

Bulkley points out that many scientists regularly contradict scientific laws in their writings to support evolutionary theory, and to dismiss creation as a laughable relic of the past. In *The Limitations of Science,* J. W. N. Sullivan wrote:

> The beginning of the evolutionary process raises a question that is as yet unanswerable. What was the origin of life on this planet? Until fairly recent times there was a pretty general belief in the occurrence of "spontaneous generation." . . . But careful experiments, notably that of Pasteur, showed that this conclusion was due to imperfect observation, and it became an accepted doctrine that life never arises except from life. So far as actual evidence goes, this is still the only possible conclusion. But since it is a conclusion that seems to lead back to some supernatural creative act, it is a conclusion that scientific men find very difficult of acceptance.[26]

In spite of the fact that life never comes from nonlife, the authors of *Science Matters* still cling to their unscientific faith. Hazen and Trefil wrote, "Life seems to have arisen in a two-step process. The first stage—chemical evolution—encompasses the origin of life from nonlife. Once life appeared, the second stage—biological evolution—took over."[27]

No scientist has ever observed life arising from nonlife, and all evidence points away from such a conclusion. "Though such scientists must be aware that they are preaching physical, chemical, and biological error," says Bulkley, "they continue to deceive the public with their 'scientific' pronouncements."[28]

To us, the wonders of the universe, of our earth, of its more than three million species, and last but not least of mankind itself, are an acknowledgment of God's existence. To us, the existence of an omnipresent God seems much less of a miracle than this Darwinian notion of chance, where "millions of years of random mixing and shuffling of molecules culminated in the appearance of one living cell."[29] This is just as logical as believing that if we put one million baboons each in front of a typewriter and then wait one million years, one of them will come up with Shakespeare's *Hamlet*. This should prove then that *Hamlet* is in no way the result of any form of creative effort, but merely the culmination of millions of years of random mixing and shuffling of letters. Nevertheless, our interest in evolution is not so much in disputing the theory of evolution as the *outcome* of this theory.

Before Darwin, there was a clear distinction between man and animal. Human behavior was looked upon as rational and animal behavior as driven by instincts. Since Darwin, man and animal have become qualitatively equal. This has lead to the idea in psychology that its salvation was to be found in the physical sciences, specifically in biology. Consequently, psychology has modeled itself on the physical sciences, which lead to the prevalence of a totally unacceptable view of man in psychology and, in fact, in all the human sciences.

Not only has evolution become a root of the "new psychology" in general, but it has also grown to become a full-fledged branch. "Evolutionary psychology," as it is called, has become a popular explanation for everything from sexual promiscuity to violent crime to ADHD. ADHD, it is said, must have had some survival value during our evolutionary history. In his book *Attention Deficit Disorder: A Different Perspective,* Hartmann proposes that ADHD traits were selected because they were valuable for the survival of the pre-agricultural human. He suggested that the traits of distractibility, impulsiveness, and even aggression would have been directly useful to a hunter. People with ADHD are, therefore, the leftovers from hunters whose ancestors evolved and matured thousands of years ago in hunting societies. Hartmann's theory, however, is debated by other scientists who relate the evolutionary development of ADHD to the so-called "fighter" and "wader" theories.[30]

These scientists have clearly forgotten the scientific principle that was advanced by Descartes some three centuries ago. This seventeenth century French philosopher stated that an allegation remains doubtful if it is based on an assumption that is still unsubstantiated.[31] This means that, *unless a theory has been substantiated, it would be unacceptable to base another theory on it.* For example, the ancient Greeks believed that the sun rises in the morning and sets in the evening because their god Helios drove a fiery chariot through the heavens. It would, however, be senseless to speculate on how many wheels his chariot might have or how many horses might draw the chariot, until the existence of Helios and his chariot have been verified. As the theory of evolution has never been verified, it is thus senseless to speculate *what* survival value ADHD might have had during our supposed evolutionary history. This amounts to no more than counting wheels and counting horses on Helios' chariot.

Perhaps Huxley was correct when he stated, "It is easy to convince men that they are monkeys. . . . The real effort lies in convincing us that we are *men*" (our italics).[32] Or perhaps, as the evolutionists claim, some brains—such as ours—have not evolved and, therefore fail to believe that men are monkeys!

The Rise of Modern Psychology

Phrenology, materialism, and the theory of evolution prepared the ground for Wundt's "new" or "modern" psychology. A confirmed materialist, a thing made sense to him and was worth pursuing only if it could be measured, quantified, and scientifically demonstrated. Seeing no way to do this with the human soul, he *denied the existence of the soul* and proposed that psychology concern itself solely with experience.[33]

Man, according to Wundt, was nothing more than a pattern of responses based upon past experience as translated through chemical experiences. His students were encouraged to examine every action and reaction of their subjects closely and attempt to measure them, and then to determine the reason for the individual differences. The focus of experimental psychology gradually turned into the physical study of the brain and central nervous system and how they respond to external stimuli. At the core of Wundt's philosophy, therefore, "was the conviction that man had no self-determinism— he could only respond to whatever the world chose to throw at him."[34]

It is important to understand the true significance of this. For centuries, man has been considered to have a free will, to be able to cause changes in his environment, and to be responsible for his actions. Wundtian theory, however, brought a gigantic shift in the traditional view of man—and one with enormous consequences. Suddenly, man was no longer thought capable of volitional control over his actions. Viewed as the product of his genetics, or viewed as constantly *affected* by his environment, his actions were thought to be preconditioned and beyond his control. In short, he became a creature at the mercy of forces around him.[35]

It is no surprise then, that religion was derided by this new and modern view. One of Wundt's students, William James—who went on to become the "Father of American Psychology"—viewed religion as not true or genuine, but deemed it therapeutic because it made the believer feel better.[36] A biographer of James, Clarence J. Karier, wrote:

> By the time James published *The Varieties of Religion* in 1902, Friedrich Nietzsche . . . has already declared, "God is dead. God remains dead. And we have killed him." With both Nietzche and James we pass from a culture with God at its center to a culture with man at its center. This fundamental shift in Western thought initiated a corresponding shift in the ideological structure of the social system. . . . Western society underwent a transformation of the basis for personal and collective values . . . Salvation was no longer a matter of survival, sin became a sickness, and such religious rituals as confession, designed to alleviate guilt and atone for sin, were replaced by individual and group psychotherapeutic interventions, designed to alleviate the guilt of anxiety neurosis.[37]

Another of Wundt's students was Emil Kraepelin, the German psychiatrist who went on to become the "Father of Psychiatry." Like his mentor, Kraepelin was a confessed materialist, seeing mental traits as hereditary and even supporting the sterilization of certain psychopaths so that the defective genes would not be passed on.[38]

But few of Wundt's pupils carried the man-is-an-animal theme as far into the spotlight as Russian physiologist and psychiatrist Ivan Pavlov did in the early twentieth century. His story is found in nearly every introductory psychology book. Pavlov and his countryman Vladimir Bekhterev—who also studied under Wundt—developed conditioned response theories through experiments on dogs.

This laid the groundwork for a fundamentally materialistic psychiatric concept which remains alive to this day, viz. that, like dogs, men are basically stimulus-response mechanisms. Furthermore, Bekhterev's and Pavlov's experiments, known as "classical conditioning," established the foundation for much of the inhuman brainwashing and mind-manipulation techniques used by the Soviet Union and China in the mid-twentieth century,[39] as well as a new field in psychology, known as *behaviorism*.

A major figure in the history of behaviorist theory is John Watson, commonly known as the father of behaviorism. John Watson expanded classical conditioning into a theory of behaviorism in which he recommended that psychology emphasize the study of overt rather than covert behavior. *Overt* behaviors are those we can observe directly, such as motor movements, speaking, and crying. *Covert* behaviors are those that only the individual who actually experiences them can observe, such as thoughts, feelings, and wishes.[40]

With covert behavior now removed from scientific study, and with the notion that man and animal are qualitatively equal, the door was opened for a new line of research—"animal psychology." Rats, as is well known, had to run through mazes in order to satisfy the curiosity of psychologists as to how learning occurs, and projections to human learning were made on this basis.

From his studies of the behavior of rats, cats, and other animals in a maze, Edward Lee Thorndike formulated his "laws of acquired behavior or learning," which he then applied to the learning of children. Thus, in 1903, *educational psychology* was born.[41] Köhler, for some reason referred to as a *child* psychologist, studied the intelligence of chimpanzees, and for many years after that time (1917) Köhler's experiments were included in discussions on learning and problem-solving processes in children.[42]

Much more recently, Harlow has carried out work with monkeys on mother-child relationships, social development, conditions in which curiosity manifests itself, "learning to learn," and the acquisition of concepts. All this was intended to throw light on human behavior. A considerable amount of work by a number of investigators has also been devoted to the study of the effects of sensory deprivation in young animals in order to better understand the effects of deprivation on cognitive development in children.[43]

Behaviorism soon became a revolutionary movement of such magnitude as to profoundly change not only the face of psychology, but also most of America's attitudinal and overt behavior:

Determinants of behavior shifted from "inner" man to "outer" man, thus giving birth to the presumption of non-accountability and non-responsibility. New methods of child rearing developed; classroom management procedures modified; legal postulates recast to accommodate new notions of "guilt," "motive," "intention," "premeditation," the emergence of "juvenile delinquency" and the "insanity plea"; and groundwork laid for changes of opinion toward homosexuality, the unwed mother, abortion, alcoholism, and other issues of morality. By 1950, the impact of behaviorism was so extensive we can but ponder the truth of Sir Walter Scott's words, "Oh, what tangled web we weave, When first we practice to deceive!"

Parents and teachers were the first to feel the brunt of behaviorism. Hundreds of child guidance clinics sprang up almost overnight to instruct parents in child rearing based on its assumptions. As behaviorism switched the responsibility for behavior from internal to external factors so did it switch the role of parents from one of authority to one of "conditioned adjustment" to the child's aggression, rudeness, need for privacy, and "rights." And because the child's behavior was considered to be symptomatic of causes within the environment, a sense of guilt was added to already frustrated parents who agonized, "Where did we go wrong?"

Teachers were likewise burdened with a sense of guilt and inadequacy. Influenced by behaviorism, educational pedagogy reversed the traditional idea of responsibility for learning from student to teacher. Non-achievement of students became the fault of teachers. To add to their stress, classrooms were bedlam. Aggressive impulses of students, freed from the restraints a sense of sin and guilt provide, became rampant. For many, the erosion of accountability served as a challenge to incite defiance. Droves of students were sent to the school counselor or referred to child psychotherapists, trained to view the word "sin" and its corollaries as possessing a quality of reproach, refrained from dealing in moral turpitude. Rather than label self-destructiveness and overt, purposeful, hurtful behavior toward others as "sin," they coined more palatable terms: "aggressive," "disruptive," "maladaptive," "antisocial." For the more serious acts which, if committed by adults would be criminal, the term "juvenile delinquency" was coined. As "juvenile delinquents," offenders were legally spared both the consequences of their behavior and the exposure of their identities. The outcome was that youth learned ways of behaving to "beat the system" of parents and teachers.[44]

The "new" view of man—that man, like the animals, is no more than a collection of genes, chemicals and stimulus-response behaviors—also laid the groundwork for ADHD, ODD, and CD. Before Wundtian theory, and especially before behaviorism, the symptoms associated with these "disorders" were viewed for what they truly are. If Johnny avoided, disliked, or was reluctant to engage in tasks that require sustained mental effort (such as his homework), and made careless mistakes in his schoolwork, a *lack* of *self-motivation* was considered to be the root of the evil. If he often fidgeted with his hands or feet, squirmed in his seat, or left the classroom when expected to remain seated, he was viewed as a child with *poor self-discipline*. If he interrupted or intruded on others, or had difficulty in awaiting his turn, the blame would fall on a *lack of self-control*. Should he defy or refuse to comply with adults' requests, he would be called *disobedient*. Aggressive, resentful, spiteful, and vindictive behaviors were signs of a *bad attitude*. Lying and stealing, straightforward, were *sins*. In short, Johnny was expected to be responsible for his actions. If he acted irresponsibly, his educators—Dad, Mom, and also his teachers—would *teach* him to be responsible.

Today, on the contrary, with behaviorism deep-rooted in Western thought, Johnny is no longer thought capable of volitional control over his actions or of deciding whether he acts in a certain way. His actions are thought to be beyond his control, affected by his heredity, so-called biochemical imbalances in the brain, food additives or even the DPT inoculation he has had as a child. His lack of self-discipline, self-control, self-motivation, disobedience, and bad attitude are thus redefined as a mental illness—ADHD, ODD, or CD.

While Johnny's future is at stake, some "expert" is filling his coffers by selling these ridiculous ideas to his—and other—parents.

Notes

1. Breggin, P. R., & Breggin, G. R., *The War Against Children of Color: Psychiatry Targets Inner-City Youth* (New York: St. Martin's Press, 1994), xvi.

2. Ibid., xvi.

3. Ibid., 96.

4. Hilts, P. J., "Scientists and their subjects debate psychiatric research ethics," *New York Times,* 1998.

5. Preller, A. C. N., *Die Wordingsweg van die Hedendaagse Psigologie. 'n Histories-wetenskapsteoretiese Beskouing* (University of Pretoria: Unpublished MA thesis, 1971).

6. "The psychiatric 'experts' cause harm," *Psychiatry Manipulating Creativity* (Los Angeles: CCHR, 1997), 42-44.

7. Skube, M., "Michael Skube on . . . Virtual pets: 'Cyberpets' symptom of society gone crazy with psychotherapy." *The Atlanta Journal and Constitution,* 27 May 1997, C02.

8. Torrey, E. F., *The Death of Psychiatry* (Radnor, PA: Little, Brown and Company, 1974), 158.

9. Masson, J. M., *Against Therapy* (New York: Atheneum, 1988), 248, cited in E. Bulkley, *Why Christians Can't Trust Psychology* (Eugene, Oregon: Harvest House Publishers, 1993), 58.

10. Collins, G. R., *Can You Trust Psychology?* (Downers Grove, IL: InterVarsity Press, 1988), 17.

11. Wiseman, B., *Psychiatry: The Ultimate Betrayal* (Los Angeles: Freedom Publishing, 1995), 6-7.

12. "Psychology as science? It's all in your mind," *Newsday,* 28 July 1994, B06.

13. Watson, J. B., & McDougall, W., *The Battle of Behaviorism: An Exposition and an Exposure* (London: Kegan Paul, Trench, Trubner & Co., Ltd., 1928), 14.

14. Heidbreder, E., *Seven Psychologies* (New York: D. Appleton-Century Publishing Co., Inc., 1933), 94.

15. Röder, T., Kubillus, V., & Burwell, A., *Psychiatrists: The Men Behind Hitler* (Los Angeles: Freedom Publishing, 1994), 228.

16. Carter, R., "Phrenological notes: Brain analysis and bumps on the head," *Independent,* 31 October 1998, 11.

17. "Bump-starting a stalled pseudo-science," *Independent,* 11 January 1997, 2.

18. Ibid.

19. Bulkley, *Why Christians Can't Trust Psychology,* 48.

20. Carter, "Phrenological notes."

21. Bulkley, *Why Christians Can't Trust Psychology,* 48.

22. Kantor, J. R., *The Scientific Evolution of Psychology* (Chicago: The Principia Press, 1969), 186, cited in Wiseman, *Psychiatry: The Ultimate Betrayal,* 8-9.

23. Wiseman, *Psychiatry: The Ultimate Betrayal,* 9.

24. Milton, R., *The Facts of Life: Shattering the Myths of Darwinism* (London: Corgi Books, 1993), 11, 294-295.

25. Noorbergen, R., *Secrets of the Lost Races* (London: New English Library, 1980), 9-11.

26. Sullivan, J. W. N., *The Limitations of Science* (New York: Mentor Books, 1933), 127, cited in Bulkley, *Why Christians Can't Trust Psychology,* 53-54.

27. Hazen, R. M., & Trefil, J., *Science Matters* (New York: Doubleday, 1990), 245, cited in Bulkley, *Why Christians Can't Trust Psychology,* 54.

28. Bulkley, *Why Christians Can't Trust Psychology,* 54.

29. Hazen & Trefil, *Science Matters,* 245, cited in Bulkley, *Why Christians Can't Trust Psychology,* 49.

30. Shelley-Tremblay, J. F., & Rosen, L. A., "Attention deficit hyperactivity disorder: An evolutionary perspective," *Journal of Genetic Psychology,* vol. 157, 1996, 443-453.

31. Frank, H. G., *Propedeùtiko de la Klerigscienco Prospektiva* (Tübingen: Gunter Narr Verlag: 1984).

32. Huxley, cited in L. Eiseley, *Darwin's Century* (Garden City: Doubleday Anchor, 1961), 182.

33. Lionni, P., & Klass, L. J., *The Leipzig Connection: The Systematic Destruction of American Education* (Portland, Oregon: Heron Books, 1980).

34. Röder, Kubillus & Burwell, *Psychiatrists: The Men Behind Hitler,* 226.

35. Lionni & Klass, *The Leipzig Connection;* Wiseman, *Psychiatry: The Ultimate Betrayal,* 10; "The beginning of the end," *Education: Psychiatry's Ruin* (Los Angeles: CCHR, 1995), 4-11.

36. Wiseman, *Psychiatry: The Ultimate Betrayal,* 10.

37. Karier, C. J., *Scientists of the Mind* (Chicago: University of Illinois

Press, 1986), 28, cited in Wiseman, *Psychiatry: The Ultimate Betrayal,* 10.

38. Wiseman, *Psychiatry: The Ultimate Betrayal,* 11.

39. Ibid.

40. Engler, B., *Personality Theories: An Introduction* (Boston: Houghton Mifflin Company, 1990), 162.

41. "Beginning of the end," *Education: Psychiatry's Ruin.*

42. Schmidt, W. H. O., *Child Development: The Human, Cultural, and Educational Context* (New York: Harper & Row, 1973), 4.

43. Ibid.

44. Idomir, L. S., *The Tangled Web. Humanism: Enrichment or Enslavement?* (Conway: Alert, 1989), 72-74.

8.

The Revolt against Morals

Since the creation of man, clear distinctions between good and bad behavior, and between right and wrong conduct have been man's guidelines for checking, judging and directing his behavior—his compass. For a great many people, this compass was the Bible.

Over the last few decades, however, white and black have become shades of gray. The rapist has become a victim of "Post Traumatic Stress Syndrome" or "Urban Stress Syndrome." The murderer has become "temporarily insane." Deviant behavior has become a product of "mental illness," ridding offenders of any moral responsibility for their actions because they are considered helpless to do anything about it. Words like ethics, morals, sin, and evil have almost disappeared from everyday usage.

Not surprisingly, with materialism and evolution as backbone, it was psychology and psychiatry who so kindly "freed" man from his "crippling burden of good and evil."[1] Since, according to evolutionary theory, there is no accountability, and according to materialism, there is no one to be accountable to, life becomes a matter of now. Why not seek the pleasures of the world?

This deliverance, however, has not caused evil to disappear or change for the better. In fact, "The repertoire of evil has never been richer," Delbanco writes. "Yet never have our responses been so weak. . . . [E]vil tends to recede into the background hum of modern life. . . . [W]e cannot readily see the perpetrator. . . . So the work of the devil is everywhere, but no one knows where to find him. . . . [W]e feel something that our culture no longer gives us the vocabulary to express."[2]

Psychology's attack on Western moral values and norms, which are to a great extent founded on Scripture, started in 1879 at Leipzig with Wilhelm Wundt. It was a natural result of materialism. If God is dead, His moral laws have no place in society. Man must therefore live according to his own rules.

To further bolster this view, we had the emergence of Freud around the turn of the twentieth century. Freud's theories, like Wundt's, call for "freedom from morality," which both men viewed as a root cause of neurosis.[3] Freud had a bitter antagonism toward religion and all forms of religious authority. He called religion the "enemy," and—almost with pleasure, it seems—predicted religion's demise in *The Future of an Illusion,* "at first only from its obsolete, offensive vestments, but then from its fundamental presuppositions as well." Here are some more examples of how he ridiculed religion in this book:

> [A] poor girl may have an illusion that a prince will come and fetch her home. It is possible; some such cases have occurred. That the Messiah will come and found a golden age is much less probable; according to one's personal attitude one will classify this belief an illusion or . . . a delusion. . . . [T]he true believer is in high degree protected against the danger of certain neurotic afflictions; by accepting the universal neurosis [meaning religion] he is spared the task of forming a personal neurosis.[4]

Wundt's and Freud's antagonism towards anything sacred were further inflamed by John Dewey, who had a profound influence on education in America and elsewhere.

Dewey, who studied under Wundt's first American student, G. Stanley Hall, implemented Wundt's view of education in the American school system, thereby claiming the title "Father of American Education."

Like Wundt, Dewey viewed children as animals requiring guidance, control, and molding, but no teaching in particular.[5] In 1928, Dewey visited the Soviet Union and wrote a series of six articles on the "wonders" of Soviet education, which had been modeled on Dewey's ideas. In her book, *Cloning of the American Mind: Eradicating Morality Through Education,* Beverly Eakman tells us:

> Students were judged on their ability to "adapt to change," for their "collective spirit," on their reactions to groups and individuals designated "enemies of the state," and on their ability to subordinate morality "to the interests of the class struggle." The family was declared a "basic form of slavery," so if the child's parents or relatives believed in God or reli-

gious morality (read *mythology*), then the student better not get caught in school. American schools adopted the same strategies beginning in the 1960s.[6]

In 1933, Dewey coauthored and signed the *Humanist Manifesto*, which was the Americanized version of the *Communist Manifesto* penned by Karl Marx. It was also signed by more than 200 signatories, of which 34 were community leaders and dignitaries.

The *Humanist Manifesto* redesigned religion, calling for a one-world "religion" which was not to be chained to "old beliefs" but to be influenced by scientific and economic change. "There is great danger of a final, and we believe fatal identification of the world religion with doctrines and methods which have lost their significance and which are powerless to solve the problem of human living in the twentieth century." Rather, religion should be a "human activity" in the direction of a "candid and explicit humanism."

A list of fifteen percepts was drafted. These included:

- Religious humanists regard the universe as self-existing and not created;
- Holding on to an organic view of life, humanists find that the traditional dualism of mind and body must be rejected;
- Humanism asserts that the nature of the universe depicted by modern science makes unacceptable any supernatural or cosmic guarantees of human values;
- We are convinced that the time has passed for theism;
- The distinction between the sacred and the secular can no longer be maintained;
- Religious Humanism considers the complete realization of human personality to be the end of man's life and seeks its development and fulfillment in the here and now; and
- Reasonable and manly attitudes will be fostered by education and supported by custom. We assume that humanism will take the path of social and mental hygiene and discourage sentimental and wishful thinking.[7]

Forty years later, in 1973, the *Humanist Manifesto II* appeared. Signed by thousands, it delivered an even more savage blow to the sanctity of religion:

As in 1933, humanists still believe that traditional theism, especially faith in the prayer-hearing God, assumed to live and care for persons, to hear and understand their prayers, and to be able to do something about them, is an unproven and outmoded faith. . . . Traditional moral codes . . . fail to meet the pressing needs of today and tomorrow. . . . Ethics is autonomous and situational needing no theological . . . sanction. . . . We strive for the good life, here and now . . . euthanasia, and the right to suicide. . . . We deplore the division of humankind on nationalistic grounds. . . . Thus we look to the development of a system of world law and a world order based upon transnational federal government.[8]

The *Humanist Manifesto* reaffirmed man's position as the center of his existence, with its attending consequences. When man became god, Heaven and Hell were replaced by here and now, and absolute values were abolished and replaced by moral relativism—right and wrong became situational and based on individual conscience. In other words, "What's right for me may be wrong for you." The result is a disrespect and disobedience for the authority of parents, man and God—"I make my own destiny," "I do my own thing," "I have my rights," "I am a free spirit," "I am not in this world to live up to your expectations."[9]

Psychiatry Helps to "Free" Man from His "Crippling Burden"

Meanwhile, while Freud and Dewey were freeing man from morality, psychiatrists were undertaking a strategy—known as the Mental Hygiene Movement—to expand their activities beyond that of caretakers of the insane to caretakers of the general public by establishing *preventive* and social work programs.[10] Prior to this, members of the profession dealt fairly exclusively with the insane. Now, psychiatry had elected for itself the task to teach people how to live properly.[11]

With the financial backing of John D. Rockefeller, whose foundations poured millions of dollars into the Mental Hygiene Movement, the development and construction of psychopathic hospitals and the training of psychiatrists, psychologists, and mental health workers across the United States, psychiatry's new vision was soon under way. The movement expanded rapidly around the globe, setting up groups in Canada, France, Belgium, England, Bulgaria, Denmark, Hungary, Czechoslovakia, Italy, Russia, Germany, Switzerland, and Australia in the 1920s. Twenty-four countries had Mental Hygiene Associations by 1930.[12]

As also happened in psychology, because it is believed to be the cause of mental illness, one preventive measure of psychiatry was to reinterpret and eventually eradicate the concepts of right and wrong. Psychiatrist G. Brock Chisholm, in an interview in 1945, stated:

> The reinterpretation and eventually eradication of the concept of right and wrong which has been the basis of child training, the substitution of intelligent and rational thinking for faith in the certainties of the old people, these are the belated objectives of practically all effective psychotherapy.

Chisholm added, "The fact is, that most psychiatrists and psychologists and many other respectable people have escaped from of these moral chains and are able to observe and think freely," and went further to say:

> We have swallowed all manner of poisonous certainties fed us by our parents, our Sunday and day school teachers, our politicians, our priests, our newspapers and others with a vested interest in controlling us. "Thou shalt become as gods, knowing good and evil," good and evil with which to keep children under control. . . with which to blind children to their glorious intellectual heritage. . . . The results, the inevitable results, are frustration, inferiority, neurosis and inability to enjoy living, to reason clearly or to make a world fit to live in.

Then he laid out the agenda for his peers: "If the race is to be freed from its crippling burden of good and evil it must be psychiatrists who take the original responsibility."[13]

By 1948, at the Third International Congress for Mental Hygiene held in London, the Mental Hygiene Movement's plans were advanced by the formation of a global organization called the World Federation for Mental Health (WFMH).[14] It was co-founded by psychiatrist J. R. Rees, a signatory of Dewey's *Humanist Manifesto*, and Chisholm.

While Chisholm had clear views on the contents of psychiatry, Rees had clear views on *how* to implement psychiatric ideas in society:

> We can therefore justifiably stress our particular point of view with regard to the proper development of the human psyche, even though our knowledge be incomplete. We must aim to make it permeate every educational activity in our

national life: primary, secondary, university and technical education ... Public life, politics and industry should all of them be within our sphere of influence. ... [W]e have made a useful attack upon a number of professions. The two easiest of them naturally are the teaching profession and the Church; the two most difficult are law and medicine. ... If we are to infiltrate the professional and social activities of other people I think we must imitate the Totalitarians and organize some kind of fifth column activity! If better ideas on mental health are to progress and spread we, as the salesmen, must lose our identity. ... Let us all, therefore, very secretly be "fifth columnists." [Fifth columnists: persons secretly aiding the enemy] ... Don't let us mention Mental Hygiene (with capital letters), though we can safely write in terms of mental health and common sense.[15]

The words of Chisholm and Rees may well have smacked of delusion, but for the fact that by the 1950s the Mental Hygiene Movement had sprawled into virtually every aspect of living.[16] Psychiatrist Walter Bromberg notes with pride,

A half century of mental hygiene effort convinced many that human behavior could indeed be modified. In the process, what had been considered 'personal' and the concern of parents, clergymen, and law enforcement agents, now became the substances of mental health programs. ... Psychiatrists talked of dealing with 'social realities' a harbinger of Community Psychiatry—the minority problem, housing, youth work, integration, social welfare, senior citizens, etc.[17]

Through their many followers, who followed their leads to the letter, Wundt's and Freud's atheistic theories were now beginning to spread rapidly to become part of everyday life. In a research study in 1976, conducted among members of the American Psychiatric Association, 95 percent reportedly acknowledged being atheists or agnostics.[18]

And although Wundt and Freud are long dead, we all share in their legacy today.

Morality Goes to Pot

In centuries past, a person came home to solace and safety. The atmosphere was one he or she created for the family, nurturing the values he or she deemed fit. There was limited outside influence to corrupt the sanctity of the home.

But things are no longer so simple. Most homes have a television. A VCR. A radio. A telephone. Many now have computers. And the wonders of our electronic age have brought us not only the world but also its dirty laundry. The TV set that once showed awed viewers live coverage of man's first steps on the moon now flashes nude flesh, bloodied bodies, and perverse messages to grown-ups and children alike. In discussing the quality of television programming, the word "wholesome" has vanished from our vocabularies. In fact, those who use it are ridiculed. . . . In the face of this assault, we react in different ways. We try to shield the children or be discriminating or perhaps we have accepted some concept that all this "life experience" is good for us and our young, that they will see it anyway, or that when it comes to morality, perhaps we need to be more open-minded. Particularly about sex. It is an incessant topic. Premarital sex. Extramarital sex. Masturbation. Homosexuality. And sexual relations between unmarried couples—once frowned upon to protect the sanctity of the family—have become heavily promoted and commonplace. It is hard to bring a video into your home that doesn't include sexual reference, language, or scene, irrelevant of story line.[19]

Few would deny that sex is an important and pleasurable part of our lives, but over the past decades the whole issue has been blown out of proportion. The new thought is clear: no sexual behavior is wrong, and those who believe sex to be restricted to wedlock are stuffy and old-fashioned. On the screen they are depicted as nerds, usually too stupid or ugly to find partners.

Sex is also being hammered into us by the print media. In the past, the hero would take the female into the bedroom, three asterisks would follow, and nine months later she would have a baby. Today, one hardly finds a novel without at least a few explicitly described sex scenes. One can open any magazine today—especially those aimed at the female readership—and one is bound to find an array of articles on relationships, pop-psych advice, sex, and more sex. As Wiseman remarks about these changed values, "One is given the distinct feeling that courtship, engagement, and marriage have given way to fleeting flings and live-ins with a string of partners, with little thought of the future."[20]

Of course, the beautiful young actors or heroes in the steamy dramas and novels never face any consequences for their sexual indulgences. No one ever has to deal with herpes, or syphilis, or chlamydia, or pelvic inflammatory disease, or infertility, or AIDS, or genital warts, or cervical cancer. No patients are ever told by a physician that there was no cure for their disease or that they would have to deal with the pain for the rest of their lives. No one ever hears that genital cancers associated with the human papilloma virus (HPV) kill more women than AIDS, or that strains of gonorrhea are now resistant to penicillin.[21]

Psychology and psychiatry have promoted the sexual dissoluteness which has become an integral part of today's society since the emergence of Sigmund Freud around the turn of the twentieth century. Without reserve, Freud wrote that "Free sexual intercourse between young males and respectable girls" was urgently necessary or society was "doomed to fall victim to incurable neuroses which reduce the enjoyment of life to a minimum, destroy the marriage relation and bring hereditary ruin on the whole coming generation."[22]

Such was the "wisdom" of Freud. His impact on the thinking of psychologists and psychiatrists internationally was summed up by Dr. Al Parides, Professor of Psychiatry at UCLA in Los Angeles, California, who said that psychiatric values had been influenced by Freud in regard to sex and in regard to morality generally. He added:

> If you look at the personal lives of all Freud's followers—his initial disciples—these people certainly have an unbelievable amount of particular problems in the sexual area. . . . The amount of deviancy as far as their sexual behavior and so forth is concerned, is enormous. If you are saying that psychiatry promotes a certain form of morality that is a deviant morality . . . yes, I would agree.[23]

Deviant indeed. Since Freud's call for free love, the promotion of promiscuity and belittlement of chastity have simply overflowed psychological and psychiatric literature. In *Escape from Childhood* (1974), the well-known John Holt, for example, advocated the overthrow of parental authority in just about every way. He advocated that children, *of whatever age*, should have the right to experience sex, drink, use drugs, drive, vote, work, own property, travel, have a guaranteed income, choose their guardians, control their learning, and have legal and financial responsibilities.[24] Gradually, this influence was foisted upon the TV, magazines, and radio—to such an extent that the media in course of time became a mere mouthpiece for psychology and psychiatry. But perhaps nowhere the promotion of this sexual liberation has had such destructive effects as it has had in the classroom, in the form of sex education. Sex education programs are now mandatory in schools in many countries.

Sex education was first introduced in Swedish schools, and was made compulsory in 1956. Since the 1950s, the claim has been made by promoters of sex education in Sweden that the program would prevent many of the problems arising out of sexual ignorance. Prostitution would be eliminated, because sex education would provide a more "natural" interrelationship between the sexes. Illegitimate births would be practically eliminated because of added knowledge about contraceptive techniques and devices. Venereal disease would be eliminated because of extensive knowledge of sexual hygiene. Divorce rates would go down because those marital problems, which were based on sexual maladjustment, would no longer be necessary.[25] However, as moral behavior results from *formation* and not from *information*, the opposite happened.

Following the introduction of compulsory sex education in Sweden, the incidence of VD and illegitimacy rose dramatically. The steady climb began the year sex education became compulsory and increased until, by 1992, 65 percent of all firstborn children were illegitimate—a nearly 450 percent increase from 1957[26]—even though half of all teenage pregnancies were aborted.[27]

The incidence of VD has increased at such an alarming rate that Sweden is today regarded as having the highest rate of VD of any civilized nation. In 1964, the reported cases were already double the figure reported in 1958. Some of the boys infected admitted to having had relations with as many as forty different girls, and 10 percent reported relations with as many as two hundred girls.[28]

The Danish record is similar. Pornography was legalized in 1967 and sex education became compulsory in 1970. Laws against homosexuality, statutory rape, and indecent exposure have been removed. In the ten years following, assault rape increased 300 percent; VD in the age group twenty and over increased 200 percent, in the sixteen to twenty age group 250 percent, and in the under fifteen age group by 400 percent. Abortions increased 500 percent, and the illegitimacy rate doubled.[29]

Despite statistics such as these, parents are still told that sex education is a good thing. William I. Bennett, writing in *The American Educator*, the journal of the American Federation of Teachers, claimed he also once favored sex education, but after examining the teaching manuals, learning kits, and guides, he has changed his mind. He now indicts the whole program along with the philosophy of the sex experts as "sleazy," "soft boiled," and "untruthful." He stated:

> One rarely, if ever, sees sex education advocates arguing for less sexual activity itself. More "responsible" activity, more "thoughtful" activity, more "well-planned out" activity, yet, but rarely if ever the simple counsel that teenagers should have less intercourse. Caution and prevention are recommended, but not restraint.[30]

Everything but restraint, he might have said. According to Mary Calderone, founder of Sex Information and Educational Council of the United States (SIECUS), which was the major force in sex education in America, "Everything that can be known about sex and sexuality, our children must have access to: masturbation, homosexuality, abortion, intercourse in film. They must begin their sexuality no later than kindergarten."[31]

At another occasion, in a lecture to adolescent boys at Blair Academy, a New Jersey prep school, she said:

> What is sex for? It's for fun . . . for wonderful sensations. . . . Sex is not something you turn off like a faucet. If you do it's unhealthy. . . . We need new values to establish when and how we should have sexual experiences. . . . You are moving beyond your parents. But you can't just move economically or educationally. You must move sexually, as well. You must learn to use sex. This is it: first, to separate yourself from your parents; second, to establish a male or female role; third, to determine value systems . . . Nobody from up on high determines this. You determine it.[32]

"The purpose of sex education is not primarily to control and suppress sex expression as in the past, but to indicate the immense possibilities for human fulfillment that human sexuality offers," said Lester Kirkendall, another SIECUS identity. "Sex must be thought of as being education, not moral indoctrination. Young people of all ages are sexual beings with sexual needs."[33]

One of the first communities to implement a SIECUS-type sex education program was Anaheim, Orange County, California. The year after the program was instituted, columnist Woodrow Palmer reported statistics in the *Santa Ana Register* showing the results:

"One class of ninth graders was taught the fundamentals of sexual relationships. This year the class graduated with exactly one half (300) of the senior girls pregnant. Another eight had to drop out in their junior year."[34]

Equally revealing are some of the statements of lesbian activist Margaret Sanger, founder of Planned Parenthood—another force in sex education in the United States—and recipient of the "Humanist of the Year" award presented by the American Humanist Association:

> Birth control appeals to the advanced radical, because it is calculated to undermine the authority of the Christian Churches. I look forward to seeing humanity free someday of the tyranny of Christianity no less than capitalism. The marriage bed is the most degenerating influence in the social order.[35]

The real shock, however, lies in the contents and materials used in some of these sex education programs. There are many more, but these should be enough to demonstrate the horrific brainwashing performed in some sex education classes:

> At a Grand Rapids, Michigan school, the local Community Mental Health Service (CMHS) provided staff to instruct 20 students in grades 7 through 11 on "Self-Pleasuring Techniques" and "Sexual Fantasies." The materials used by the instructors included graphic descriptions of masturbation as well as oral and group sex. Parents were forced to file a suit against the school and the CMHS.

> In the fifth grade "health" class in Lincoln City, Oregon, homosexuality was presented to 11-year-olds as an alternative lifestyle. Anal intercourse was described. In the same class, a plastic model of female genitalia with a tampon insert was passed around to the boys to encourage their understanding of tampons. Birth controls were also passed around and explained.[36]

An "AIDS Quiz," given to [German] children from twelve years of age and which also has a multiple choice answer to check, asks, "In which situation could you be infected by AIDS?" Answer "G" says: "By swallowing sperm?"[37]

And here are a few quotations from a book by Pomeroy, *Boys and Sex*, an Australian guide to sex education:

> Those who have made the decision to have intercourse have

the further responsibility of exercising their ingenuity in finding the best place to have it—some available spot where the
chances of discovering are not great. . . . Sometimes the couple
uses the home of either the male or female, which is fine if
they can be absolutely sure that the parents won't return
home unexpectedly (p. 134). . . . There is essentially nothing
that humans do sexually that is abnormal, even homosexuality would be almost normal because so many boys are
involved in it (p. 147). I have known cases of farm boys who
have had a loving sexual relationship with an animal and felt
good about their behavior until they got to college, where
they learned for the first time that what they had done was
"abnormal." [Pomeroy's] advice is to keep the activity a secret
to avoid ridicule (p. 149).[38]

Isn't this absolutely horrifying? Yet, this is precisely what happens if God is discredited and man consequently places himself in
the center. As Dr. Edmund Leach, an anthropologist, wrote in an
incredibly galling article in *The Saturday Evening Post*, November
1968, entitled "We scientists have a right to play God":

There can be no source for these moral judgements except
the scientist himself. In traditional religion, morality was
held to derive from God, but God was only credited with
the authority to establish and enforce moral rules because he
was also credited with supernatural powers of creation and
destruction. Those powers have now been usurped by man.[39]

What Dr. Leach has not discovered yet is that man suffers
adverse consequences when he defies God's moral laws. Western
civilization will not be the first to pluck the fruits of immorality. J.
D. Unwin, a British social anthropologist, who spent seven years
studying the births and deaths of eight civilizations, concluded that
every known culture in the world's history has followed the same
pattern: during its early days of existence, premarital and extramarital sexual relationships were strictly prohibited. Apparently this in-
hibition of sexual expression leads to great creative energy, causing
the culture to prosper. Much later in the life of the society, its people
began to rebel against the strict prohibitions, demanding the freedom to release their internal passions. As the mores weakened, the
social energy abated, eventually resulting in the decay or destruction
of the civilization. Dr. Unwin stated that the energy which holds a
society together is sexual in nature. When a man is devoted to one
woman and one family, he is motivated to build, save, protect, plan,

and prosper on their behalf. However, when his sexual interests are dispersed and generalized, his effort is invested in the gratification of sexual desires.[40]

Maybe we should heed to the warnings of the prophet Isaiah to God's chosen people in bondage, the consequence of their turning away from Him to pursue pagan idols (Isa. 5:20-21): "Woe to those who call evil good and good evil, who put darkness for light and light for darkness, who put bitter for sweet and sweet for bitter. Woe to those who are wise in their own eyes and clever in their own sight."

Creating a Drug Culture

A 1995 Columbia University survey showed that 67 percent of the adults, and 76 percent of the 12- to 17-year-olds questioned, agreed that pop culture—TV, movies, magazines, and music—encouraged the use of illegal drugs.[41]

Few people know the history of how the drug culture has become part of our everyday lives. As already stated, the social problems of drugs were relatively narrow and confined until the 1950s. But since then, the situation has changed drastically.

One of the turning points came in 1954 with the introduction of Thorazine. For the first time, a psychotropic (mind-altering) drug was in wide use. Around the same time, another drug was gaining steady popularity. It was called LSD.[42]

After the discovery of LSD in 1943, psychiatrist Werner Stoll was one of the first to investigate and map out how the drug could be used for psychological purposes. Enthusiastically received by other psychiatrists in the 1950s, LSD became the perfect vehicle for psychiatry to promote the concept of improving life through recreational psychotropic drugs.[43] It was not long before America's intelligence agency, the CIA, took an interest in LSD. One of D. Ewen Cameron's pet projects—he worked for the CIA in the 1950s—involved the use of drugs, electric shocks, and hypnosis to wipe out a person's memory and to implant new ones. Under his guidance, a British psychiatrist and visiting professor of psychiatry conducted experiments on 24 different patients.[44]

The CIA soon began to fund psychiatric researchers who were working with the drug. One of these was Dr. Harris Isbell of the Kentucky Addiction Research Center in Lexington. Despite its name, the Center was actually a penitentiary for heroin addicts, sexual deviants, and the mentally ill. It was also, along with fourteen other secret penal and mental institutions, the place where the CIA sent drugs to be tested. Like the Nazi psychiatrists of World War II, Isbell used his prisoners—exclusively African-American—as guinea pigs, experimenting with over eight hundred compounds the CIA sent him over the course of ten years.[45] In one chilling experiment, Isbell kept seven men on LSD for seventy-seven days. The brutality of these experiments is clearly illustrated by cases such as that of a 19-year-old, who, after taking LSD once, claimed that he had hallucinated and suffered for sixteen or seventeen hours.[46] In exchange for their cooperation, Isbell would give his "patients" as much heroin or morphine as they wanted. In fact, "it became an open secret among street junkies that if the supply got tight, you could always commit yourself to Lexington."[47] Other psychiatrists followed the same line of action, testing LSD in every possible and impossible way, often combining it with psychotherapy.

In the mid-1950s, psychiatrist Dr. Oscar Janiger lured writers, musicians, actors and filmmakers into taking LSD. As opinion leaders, these individuals were capable of greatly influencing the values and trends in society.[48] By the late 1950s, LSD had virtually become a buzzword in Hollywood circles as movie stars were given their first trips by their psychiatrists. Lee and Shlain tell us, "psychiatrists who practiced LSD were inundated with inquiries."[49] Books, motion pictures, and journal programs chanted the healing powers of LSD. Notably, *LIFE* magazine, whose publisher Henry Luce tried the drug, ran articles promoting it. A March 1963 article claimed that LSD was "derived from a *natural* product." And by the turbulent 1960s, LSD had become the symbol for New Age thinking and living.[50]

With his slogan of "turn on, tune in, and drop out," Timothy Leary, a professor in clinical psychology at Harvard, inspired a whole generation of college students in the mid-1960s to experiment with LSD and other psychedelic substances. Through magazine interviews, television appearances, movies, records, and books, Leary projected himself as a culture hero of a new generation fighting for the individual's rights to alter his own consciousness—a right which Leary maintained was guaranteed by the Constitution of the United States.[51]

LSD was also popular among so-called "legitimate" researchers. Lauretta Bender, a psychiatrist at Creedmore State Hospital in New

York, tested the effects of LSD on autistic and schizophrenic children. In a workshop, organized by the psychopharmacology branch of the National Institute of Mental Health, she summarized the effect of LSD on eighty-nine children as follows:

> We gave this [LSD] first to young, autistic children, and we found we were able to get an improvement in their general well-being, general tone, habit patterning, eating patterns and sleeping patterns. . . . We also tried LSD on two adolescent boys who were mildly schizophrenic. . . . They became disturbed to the extent that they said we were experimenting on them. . . . We . . . have found that it [LSD] is one of the most effective methods of treatment we have for childhood schizophrenia.[52]

By 1968, LSD, marijuana, and cocaine were available on street corners and schoolyards throughout America. But the deleterious effects of LSD—overdoses, bad trips, "burned-out brains," a plummet in sexual values, and personal responsibility—were now also becoming clear. The drug revolution "racked nations and families around the world."[53] When the psychedelic revolution was furthermore "turning people out" to such a degree that they were actively protesting the Vietnam War and demanding social reforms, the CIA eventually withdrew the LSD and all of its derivatives completely from the market.[54]

But it was too late. Once LSD vanished, the market became glutted with heroin. The American drug culture was now firmly established, and, as the years passed, it found its way to the grade school playgrounds, and from there it spread over the rest of the Western world. The drug market, firmly established with the aid of psychiatrists, now opened up a new market for psychiatrists—the *rehabilitation* of drug addicts:

> This necessitated more facilities, more research—and much more money. After all, panic-stricken Americans demanded it; now there were "drug crazies" everywhere who had previously been hidden behind the doors of large mental institutions. Now any normal-looking person could suddenly go psychotic at any time—and drugs and addicts were everywhere on the streets. Taking advantage of the situation, the psychiatric community could now attempt to handle the "runaway insanity" to which they had contributed so richly.

"Give us your money," they said in essence, "and we will make it go away."[55]

But the psychiatric community clearly did not really want to remove drugs from our society. While national campaigns against illegal drug abuse were set in motion, psychiatry continued to promote drug use in legal form. Within eight months after Thorazine hit the market in 1954, it had been given to an estimated two million patients.[56] So powerful was the drug that one of its leading researchers, Heinz E. Lehmann, promoted it as "a pharmacological substitute for lobotomy."[57] The public's resistance to the drug was warded off with the argument that it is okay to give psychotropic drugs to mental patients, since they are mentally ill. But it did not take long before the idea was fixed that drugs could also be administered for minor problems, and finally, also to the perfectly normal.[58]

In 1960, Librium, a tranquilizer, appeared on pharmacy shelves, and, in 1963, Valium, another tranquilizer, was introduced. Valium became the most prescribed drug in medical history, and remained at the top of the drug hit parade until about 1984, when its curses—addiction and side effects—became known.[59] By 1973, only nineteen years after the introduction of Thorazine, about a third of Americans had taken some form of psychiatric drug.[60] In 1981, Xanax came on the market—a drug that would later be connected to violent episodes in some users[61]—and in 1987, we experienced the emergence of Prozac. Despite 160 lawsuits brought against its manufacturer for alleged violent or suicidal reactions, psychiatrists continued to prescribe the drug in record quantities. In 1988, sales hit $125 million; in 1989, $350 million, and in 1993, $1.2 billion.[62] Despite the fact that no adequate research has yet been done on the desirability of such a practice, Prozac is also increasingly prescribed to children. According to IMS America, a company that tracks prescriptions and the sale of drugs, doctors prescribed or recommended Prozac and similar drugs like Zoloft and Paxil 1.27 million times for youngsters aged ten to nineteen in 1995, up from 696,000 in 1993. For children aged three to nine, the number in 1995 was 59,000, up from 36,000 in 1994.[63]

In a retrospective appraisal of his profession, psychiatrist Walter

Afield said, "People my age and older, who are very senior, who have been through this whole thing say, 'Dear God, what have we done?' "[64]

Notes

1. Chisholm, G. B., "The reestablishment of peacetime society"—The William Alanson White memorial lectures, 1945, published in *Psychiatry: Journal of the Biology and the Pathology of Interpersonal Relations*, vol. 9(1), February 1946, 3-11.

2. Delbanco, A., *The Death of Satan*, 1995, cited in "A letter of hope," *Psychiatry Destroying Religion* (Los Angeles: CCHR, 1997), 2-3.

3. "The progressive dismantling of a workable education system." *Psychiatry: Betraying and Drugging Children* (Los Angeles: CCHR, 1998), 4-7.

4. Freud, S., *The Future of an Illusion* (New York: W. D. Robson-Scott, 1953).

5. "The progressive dismantling of a workable education system," *Psychiatry: Betraying and Drugging Children*.

6. Eakman, B. K., *Cloning of the American Mind: Eradicating Morality through Education* (Lafayette: Huntington House Publishers, 1998), 135.

7. *Humanist Manifesto I,* http://www.jeremiahproject.com/prophecy/manifesto1.html

8. *Humanist Manifesto II,* http://www.geocities.com/Athens/6276/manifest2.html

9. Idomir, L. S., *The Tangled Web. Humanism: Enrichment or Enslavement?* (Conway: Alert, 1989), 89-90.

10. "Psychology: Eradicating souls," *Psychiatry: Destroying Religion* (Los Angeles: CCHR, 1997), 8-17.

11. Wiseman, B., *Psychiatry: The Ultimate Betrayal* (Los Angeles: Freedom Publishing, 1995), 70-71.

12. Ibid., 72, 74.

13. Chisholm, "The reestablishment of peacetime society."

14. Wiseman, *Psychiatry: The Ultimate Betrayal*, 77.

15. Rees, J. R., "Strategic planning for Mental Health," *Mental Health*, vol. 1(4), 103-106, cited in Wiseman, *Psychiatry: The Ultimate Betrayal*,

77-78.

16. Wiseman, *Psychiatry: The Ultimate Betrayal,* 78.

17. Bromberg, W., *From Shaman to Psychotherapist* (Chicago: Henry Regnery Co.), 107, cited in Wiseman, *Psychiatry: The Ultimate Betrayal,* 78.

18. Larson, D. B., et al., "Systematic analysis of research on religious variables in four major psychiatric journals," *The American Journal of Psychiatry,* vol. 143(3), March 1986, 329-334, cited in Wiseman, *Psychiatry: The Ultimate Betrayal,* 13.

19. Wiseman, *Psychiatry: The Ultimate Betrayal,* 22-23.

20. Ibid., 25.

21. Dobson, J., *The New Dare to Discipline* (Wheaton, Illinois: Tyndale House Publishers, Inc., 1992), 214.

22. Thornton, E. M., *The Freudian Fallacy* (New York: The Dial Press, 1984), 144-145.

23. "Psychology: Eradicating souls," *Psychiatry: Destroying Religion.*

24. Dobson, J., *The Strong-Willed Child* (Eastbourne: Kingsway Publications, 1993), 160.

25. Brodin & Rowe, *America's Sex Education Furore* (Canada, 1975) cited in J.M. Wallis, *Chaos in the Classroom* (Bullsbrook: Veritas Publishing Company Pty. Ltd., 1984), 243.

26. "Psychiatry eradicates morals," *Psychiatry Destroying Religion* (Los Angeles: CCHR, 1997), 54-61.

27. Wallis, J. M., *Chaos in the Classroom* (Bullsbrook: Veritas Publishing Company Pty. Ltd., 1984), 247.

28. *Sex Education and the Schools,* May 1979, cited in Wallis, *Chaos in the Classroom,* 247.

29. Ibid.

30. Bennett, W. I., *The National Educator,* September 1981, cited in Wallis, *Chaos in the Classroom,* 274.

31. *Western Voice,* 13 February 1969, cited in Wallis, *Chaos in the Classroom,* 244.

32. *Look,* 8 March 1966, cited in Wallis, *Chaos in the Classroom,* 245.

33. "Sex Education," SIECUS Discussion Guide, cited in Wallis, *Chaos in the Classroom,* 243.

34. Wallis, *Chaos in the Classroom*, 248

35. "The Humanist Manifesto harms religion. Psychology redefines religion," *Psychiatry Destroying Religion* (Los Angeles: CCHR, 1997), 14-15.

36. "Meddling with minds," *Education: Psychiatry's Ruin* (Los Angeles: CCHR, 1995), 16-21.

37. "Psychiatry eradicates morals," *Psychiatry Destroying Religion.*

38. Pomeroy, W. B., *Boys and Sex* (Harmondsworth: Penguin Books, 1968), 134-149.

39. Leach, E., "We scientists have the right to play God," *Saturday Evening Post,* November 1968, cited in Dobson, *The Strong-Willed Child,* 215.

40. Dobson, J., *Dare to Discipline* (Toronto: Bantam Books, 1977), 146-147.

41. "Pop culture and drugs," *Wall Street Journal,* 26 February 1995.

42. Wiseman, *Psychiatry: The Ultimate Betrayal,* 218.

43. "LSD: Psychiatry controlling culture," *Psychiatry Manipulating Creativity* (Los Angeles: CCHR, 1997), 22-25.

44. Röder, T., Kubillus, V., & Burwell, A., *Psychiatrists: The Men Behind Hitler* (Los Angeles: Freedom Publishing, 1994), 281.

45. Ibid., 284.

46. Wiseman, *Psychiatry: The Ultimate Betrayal,* 100.

47. Lee, M. A., & Shlain, B., *Acid Dreams* (New York: Grove Press, Inc., 1985), 24, cited in Röder, Kubillus & Burwell, *Psychiatrists: The Men Behind Hitler,* 284.

48. "LSD: Psychiatry controlling culture," *Psychiatry Manipulating Creativity.*

49. Lee & Shlain, *Acid Dreams,* cited in Wiseman, *Psychiatry: The Ultimate Betrayal,* 220.

50. "LSD: Psychiatry controlling culture," *Psychiatry Manipulating Creativity.*

51. Bowart, W., *Operation Mind Control* (New York: Dell Publishing Co., 1978), 79.

52. Bender, L., "LSD and amphetamine in children," in D. H. Efron (ed.), *Psychotomimetic Drugs* (New York: Raven Press, 1969), cited in

Röder, Kubillus & Burwell, *Psychiatrists: The Men Behind Hitler*, 285.

53. Wiseman, *Psychiatry: The Ultimate Betrayal*, 222.

54. Röder, Kubillus & Burwell, *Psychiatrists: The Men Behind Hitler,* 285.

55. Ibid., 286.

56. Swazey, J. P., *Chlorpromazine in Psychiatry* (Massachusetts Institute of Technology, 1974), 160.

57. Lehmann, H. E., "Therapeutic results with Chlorpromazine," *Canadian Medical Association Journal,* vol. 72, 1955, cited in Wiseman, *Psychiatry: The Ultimate Betrayal,* 196.

58. Wiseman, *Psychiatry: The Ultimate Betrayal,* 197-198.

59. Rosenblatt, S. & Dodson, R., *Beyond Valium: The Brave New World of Psychochemistry* (New York: Putnam's Sons, 1981), 45.

60. Bernstein, A., & Lennard, H. L., "The American way of drugging," *Society,* vol. 10(4), May/June 1973, 14, cited in Wiseman, *Psychiatry: The Ultimate Betrayal,* 198.

61. Wiseman, *Psychiatry: The Ultimate Betrayal,* 199.

62. Ibid.

63. "Cry the poor little pill poppers," *The Star,* 1996.

64. Wiseman, *Psychiatry: The Ultimate Betrayal,* 223.

9.

Chaos in the Classroom

The whole teaching-and-learning continuum, which was once tied in an orderly and productive way to the passing of generations and the growth of the child into a man—this whole process has exploded in our faces.[1]

Although there is widespread agreement that something is drastically wrong with Western education, few people know who or what to blame. The educational establishment's excuse for the failure to educate children is usually that they need more money. This, however, is a weak excuse. In America, for example, taxpayers have increased education spending by 225 percent since 1960 (allowing for inflation), when the SAT scores started to decline.[2] This excuse becomes especially weak when one compares the results achieved by American students with those achieved by the Japanese in the 1980s, whose per-pupil expenditure was far less than the United States.

In 1983, the same year in which the National Commission on Excellence in Education declared America to be a "nation at risk," Thomas Rohlen's book, *Japan's High Schools*, was published. Comparing the American and Japanese educational standards, the author concluded that the Japanese high school diploma was arguably the equivalent of a U.S. bachelor's degree. "I found this conclusion hard to believe at first," he wrote. "But the more I looked at the fundamental facts, the more convinced I became that the majority of high school graduates in Japan would compare well with our university graduates in terms of basic knowledge in all fields and in mathematics and in science skills."[3] Yet, despite a much more challenging school curriculum, Japan succeeded in leading fully 91 percent of their students through high school in the 1980s, while only 75 percent of U.S. high school students managed to graduate.[4] And the last sobering piece of news which should silence requests for more money is that Japan averaged forty-one students per class, compared to twenty-six for the United States, and the overall per-pupil expenditure in Japan was 50 percent less than that in the United States.[5]

To find the culprits of the literacy crisis and the collapse in standards of education, one simply has to turn the clock back to the beginning of the twentieth century when psychology and psychiatry—in the words of psychiatrist Ralph Truitt—started their "attack" on the educational system.[6] The place is the Department of Psychology at Columbia University's Teachers College in New York.

Beginning of the Rising Tide of Mediocrity

At the time of the development of his "educational psychology," Edward Lee Thorndike was a staff member at the above-mentioned Teachers College. The first task of educational psychology was to eliminate the education fundamentals of reading and writing and redefine education into psychological or psychiatric contexts. Thorndike stated his aspirations in a book he coauthored in 1929:

> Despite rapid progress in the right direction, the program of the average elementary school is too narrow and academic in character. Traditionally, the elementary school has been primarily devoted to teaching the fundamental subjects, the three R's, and closely related disciplines. . . . Artificial exercises, like drills on phonics, multiplication tables, and formal writing movements, are used to a wasteful degree. Subjects such as arithmetic, language, and history include content that is intrinsically of little value. Nearly every subject is enlarged unwisely to satisfy the academic ideal of thoroughness. . . . Elimination of the unessential by scientific study, then, is one step in improving the curriculum.[7]

It is strange that anybody would have wanted to improve the American curriculum in the early twentieth century. High standards of classroom conduct were maintained. Students were well versed in history, the arts, and in classical literature. The three R's—reading, 'riting, and 'rithmetic—were emphasized. Children were sent to school to learn—period. In 1910, the literacy rate was so high it was predicted that "the public schools will in a short time practically eliminate illiteracy."[8] Notwithstanding, with his "animal psychology" as background, Thorndike started pouring out his new educational ideas on how the curriculum should be improved. In fact, he published 507 books, monographs, and articles on the subject.

Like all followers of Wundt, Thorndike did not see humans as self-willed, capable of choice and decision, but as stimulus-response mechanisms. In *The Principles of Teaching Based on Psychology* he defined teaching as "the art of giving and withholding stimuli with the result of producing or preventing certain responses." (In this definition, the term stimulus is used widely for any event which influences a person, for a word spoken to him, a look, a sentence which he reads, the air he breathes, etc. The term response is used for any reaction made by him, a new thought, a feeling of interest, a bodily act, any mental or bodily condition resulting from the stimulus.) "The aim of the teacher," Thorndike said, "is to produce desirable and prevent undesirable changes in human beings by producing and preventing certain responses."[9] Thorndike made the role of the teacher sound like that of the animal trainer.

Disguised as "educational psychology," Thorndike's "animal psychology" soon began to leave its mark on education. His role in educational "improvement," however, was soon to be exceeded by that of John Dewey, who joined Thorndike at Teachers College. Dewey—who later coauthored the *Humanist Manifesto*—was one of the founders of the philosophical school of pragmatism, and set the ball rolling for an amalgam of educational psychology and socialism. It became known as "progressive education." Emanating from the Columbia College, it slowly but surely became commonplace in U.S. schools and in schools of other Western countries.[10]

Pragmatism is a philosophy based on evolution. It rejects the idea of a spiritual being and creationism, believing that the universe, with man as part of it, is in a process of evolving, having no beginning or end. Man's authority is his *experience*. There is no ultimate or absolute truth. Truth is always tentative, can only be derived from human experience, and can be modified or rejected by future experiences.[11] Absolute norms for behavior, therefore, do not exist. Man must adapt himself to the demands of the environment. Furthermore, the pragmatist absolutizes a "practice that works." To find this "practice that works," the pragmatist will throw all principles overboard, as long as certain practical ends can be achieved. According to the pragmatist "the end justifies the means."[12] Applied to education, the curriculum, and teaching methods must be tried, rejected, revised or adapted, as the situation warrants.[13]

Based on the philosophy of pragmatism, progressive education elevated practical experience above formal learning such as reading, writing and math, which is often accompanied by drilling, and vocational training above traditional disciplines. *What* children learned, according to Dewey, was not as important as *how* they learned. Denying the existence of overarching, universal truths, he said that schools shouldn't teach facts. Instead, they should teach a *process of inquiry*. In a process-oriented history class, Johnny doesn't learn the key events of the founding of a nation. Instead, he grinds corn so he can experience how the Indians lived. In a process-oriented science class, Johnny doesn't learn the basic facts of biology. He writes an essay on how it would feel to be a groundhog. In social studies, Johnny doesn't learn the facts of geography and culture. Instead, he reads a story about a family living in some Third World village, in order to get a feeling of their way of life.[14]

These progressive methods assumed that children would develop the skills they required through a few carefully arranged direct experiences. This placed a great deal of trust in the child's ability to learn general skills without any informational knowledge from which to work. It was a trust that was later shown to be misplaced.

Dewey accused the educators of his day of being "cultists" because of their view that "the first three years of a child's school life ought to be taken up with learning to read and write in his own language." "The true way," Dewey countered, "is to teach them incidentally, as an outgrowth of . . . social activities [since] language is not primarily an expression of thought, but a means of communication."[15]

Dewey's was an extremely radical idea (that language is not an expression of thought). The biblical view, for example, is precisely the opposite: what comes out of a person's mouth is the measure of what is inside his heart.[16]

With large-scale financial support of inter alia oil tycoon John D. Rockefeller, progressive education made its debut into American public schools in the 1920s.[17] From there it spread to other countries. "Progressive education" soon became a target of numerous and widespread critique, being blamed for the failure of students in math and science, and the disintegration of classroom discipline. So-called open *laissez faire* schools tested Dewey's "process of inquiry" to the limit:

> We had certain hours allotted to various subjects but we were free to dismiss anything that bored us. In fact, it was school policy that we were forbidden to be bored or miserable or made to compete with one another. There were no tests and no hard times. When I was bored with math, I was excused and allowed to write short stories in the library. The

way we learned history was by trying to recreate its least
important elements. One year, we pounded corn, made te-
pees, ate buffalo meat and learned two Indian words. That
was early American history. Another year we made elaborate
costumes, clay pots, and paper-mache gods. That was Greek
culture. Another year we were all maidens and knights in
armor because it was time to learn about the Middle Ages.
We drank our orange juice from tinfoil goblets but never
found out what the Middle Ages were. They were just "The
Middle Ages. . . ."

We spent great amounts of time being creative because we
had been told by our incurably optimistic mentors that the
way to be happy in life was to create. Thus, we didn't learn
to read until we were in the third grade because early reading was thought to discourage creative spontaneity. The one
thing they taught us very well was to hate intellectuality and
anything connected with it. . . . What we did do was to continually form and reform interpersonal relationships and that's
what we thought learning was all about and we were happy.

The happiness, however, did not last for long:

When we finally were graduated from Canaan, however, all
the happy little children fell down the hill. We felt a profound sense of abandonment. So did our parents. After all
that tuition money, let alone the loving freedom, their children faced high school with all the glorious prospects of the
poorest slum-school kids. And so it came to be. No matter
what school we went to, *we* were the underachievers and the
culturally disadvantaged.

For some of us, real life was too much—one of my oldest
friends . . . killed himself two years ago after flunking out of
the worst high school in New York at 20. Various others
have put in time in mental institutions where they were free,
once again, to create during occupational therapy.

During my own high school years, the school psychologist
was baffled by my lack of substantive knowledge. He suggested to my mother that I be given a battery of psychological tests to find out why I was blocking out information. The
thing was, I wasn't blocking because I had no information to
block. . . . The parents of my former classmates can't figure
out what went wrong. They had sent in bright curious chil-

dren and gotten back, nine years later, helpless adolescents. . . . Now I see my 12-year-old brother (who is in a traditional school) doing college-level math and I know that he knows more about many other things besides math than I do. And I also see traditional education working in the case of my 15-year-old brother. . . .[18]

According to Blumenfeld, Dewey's purpose with "progressive education" was to erode literacy standards. Dewey was a fanatical socialist, and considered high literacy to be incompatible with his social goals:

> To Dewey, the greatest enemy of socialism was the private consciousness that seeks knowledge in order to exercise its own individual judgement and authority. High literacy gave the individual the means to seek knowledge independently. To Dewey it created and sustained the individual system which was detrimental to the social spirit needed to build a socialist society.[19]

Unfortunately, many influential educators followed in Dewey's footsteps, adapting their methods to suit their own selfish ends. In time, in the words of Blumenfeld, "public education became nothing more but a shoddy, fraudulent piece of goods sold to the public at an astronomical price."[20]

"Affective" Education Replaces "Intellectual" Education

Dewey had opened the door for other professional educators to apply pressure for the replacement of traditional disciplines with nonacademic courses. One of these influential figures was a psychologist by the name of Carl Rogers. In 1924, Rogers went to Union Theological Seminary, but after two years moved to Teachers College, Columbia University, where he was exposed to the Thorndikean behavioral approaches, Dewey's philosophical school of pragmatism, and the Freudian orientation of the Institute for Child Guidance, where he had an internship. In 1931, he received his Ph.D. from Columbia University and in 1939 he published his first book, entitled *The Clinical Treatment of the Problem Child.*[21]

Rogers disagreed with Freud's dark, pessimistic and largely negative picture of personality, as well as the limited picture of the person as a machine or robot that emerged from behaviorism.[22] According to Rogers, man can take charge of his own life and can go beyond or transcend his existing circumstances. He can shape himself, redesign himself, and make himself into whatever likeness he chooses. He chooses whatever he thinks is best for him.[23]

The philosophy underlying these ideas is called *existentialism*. Because self-actualization is the goal of existentialism, morals are viewed as prohibiting, restricting and confining and must be discarded. The aim of existentialism is to free, to liberate from the "thou shalt nots;" to make choices based not on the "realities that come to us through traditional system-building," but on the "virgin stuff of reality" residing within the self: "*human experiences in its raw form.*"[24]

With this philosophy as background, Rogers urged teachers to be non-judgmental, to "humanize" the classroom, to raise the self-esteem of students.[25] The teacher must be a facilitator. In the words of Rogers, the "teacher does not set lesson tasks. He does not assign readings. He does not lecture or expound, unless requested to. He does not evaluate and criticize, unless the student wishes his judgement on a product. He does not give examinations. He does not set grades."[26]

According to Rogers, no one should ever be trying to learn something for which he sees no *relevance*. The student should be asked: "What do you want to learn? What things puzzle you? What are you curious about? What issues concern you? What problems do you wish you could solve?"[27]

The fact that he has neither foreknowledge of the material to be learned, nor experience in its application in the real world beyond the walls of the school, should not be seen as a stumbling block. At the heart of the relevance notion, precisely, is the belief that current *emotional responses* are a reliable guide to the future usefulness or meaningfulness of education.[28] As Carl Rogers said, the man who would "do what 'felt right' in this immediate moment" would "find this in general to be a trustworthy guide to his behavior."[29] If emotions were indeed so prescient and virtually omniscient, then of course there would be little reason to rely on experience—which must mean the experience of others, in the case of inexperienced students.[30]

As Sowell remarks, it is hard to imagine how a small child first learning the alphabet can appreciate the full implications of learning these particular twenty-six abstract symbols in an arbitrarily fixed order. Yet his lifelong access to the intellectual treasures of centuries depends on his mastery of these symbols. His ability to organize and retrieve innumerable kinds of information from sources ranging from encyclopedias to computers depends on his having memorized that purely arbitrary order. There is not the slightest reason in the world why a small child should be expected to grasp the significance of all this. Instead, he learns these symbols and their order because his parents and teachers want him to learn them—not because he sees its "relevance."[31] Similarly, there are many other things that a child has to learn, even though he cannot himself see the relevance or the meaning. He simply learns them because his educators (parents and teachers) have the insight to know how important these will be for his future.

The consequence of this romantic vision, however, was that curricula were redesigned to suit the current emotional appeal of students. Education was no longer assessed in terms of its future rewards, but in terms of the "excitement" it held for students.[32] The pendulum has swung completely from the one extreme to the other, from the ideas of John Locke that instruction should be difficult, uninteresting, not pleasurable and should consist of drill because only then would it have value, to the idea that instruction should equal entertainment.

Rogers also said that children must be encouraged to air their views and their views must be taken seriously, because that will improve their self-image. It does not matter whether their views make any sense or not, because opinions cannot be right or wrong. Briefly stated, Rogers replaced "intellectual education" with "affective education." The phrase "I feel" became the way whereby American students introduced a conclusion, rather than "I think," or "I know," much less "I conclude."[33]

By the mid-1970s, education's high priests had finally succeeded in their long-standing struggle (since the heydays of Edward Lee Thorndike and John Dewey) to shift schools away from academics and scholarship to socialization and guardianship:

> Teachers threw out stuffy old books, learned how to say "Hey, Man!", exchanged their dresses and suits for blue jeans, and dismissed "the value of *x*." Likewise, students' dress codes and rote learning were scrapped, tests and curricula were dumbed down, once-neat rows of desks were traded for "open classrooms," teacher lecturing and grading scales were condemned, and a technique called "behavioral conditioning" . . . began replacing drill and repetition.[34]

Making Our "Sick" Children Well

A further "contribution" of Rogers to education was that he cooperated with other psychologists and psychiatrists to create programs that were aimed at changing the values, attitudes and beliefs of children. Their programs were supposed *to help children to choose for themselves what they believed and to establish their own values.* The reason why "self-chosen" values were essential was summarized in 1973 by psychiatrist Chester M. Pierce. In an address to the Childhood International Educational Seminar, he claimed, "Every child in America entering the school at the age of five is insane because he comes to school with certain allegiances to our founding Fathers, toward his parents, toward a belief in a supernatural being, toward the sovereignty of this nation as a separate entity." Then he laid out the agenda for his colleagues saying, "It is up to you [psychologists and psychiatrists] to make these sick children well—by creating the international child of the future."[35]

One of the "lifeboats" that was to save children from their moralizing parents and their allegiances toward them, was values clarification, a psychological method that was introduced in American schools in the 1970s. In essence, it is a humanistic process of reasoning which was incorporated in all segments of social education—"death education," "survival education," "drug education," "sex education," "peace education," etc.

In his book, *Attack on the Family*, James Robinson describes values clarification in action:

> Under the "Values Clarification" method, the dynamics of the situation exerts immense pressure on the child to abandon previous values, wherever derived, and replace them with new ones. The system coaxes the child to lay bare his heart, mind and soul before his teacher and his peers. In the discussion that follows, his personal convictions and feelings are subject to comment and ridicule. If he is challenged, he must defend his values and the way he arrived at them. If his choice of value can be traced to parents, church, or any other source, it is automatically disqualified under the "rules of the game," which say the only valid values are self-chosen. This exposes the child who has been taught obedience and respect for parents to a cruel brand of intimidation. Skillful Humanist teachers can manipulate discussions so as to make peer pressure so intense that few children are strong enough to

adhere to their parent-taught values at all. Those who do so can hardly escape feelings of shame and ostracism.[36]

Among the questions used to discredit parents and undermine parent-taught values are:

- What disturbs you most about your parents?
- Would you bring up your children differently from the way you are being brought up?
- What would you change?
- As a child, did you ever run away from home?
- Did you ever want to?
- Who is the "boss" in your family?
- Do you believe in God?
- How do you feel about homosexuality?

In addition to questions, students have an "opportunity" to tell things, such as:

- Tell where you stand on the topic of masturbation.
- Reveal who in your family brings you the greatest sadness, and why. Then share who brings you the greatest joy.
- Tell some ways in which you will be a better parent than your own parents are now.
- Tell something about a frightening sexual experience.[37]

Another values clarification handbook has blanks to fill in, such as:

- Someone in my family who really gets me angry is

  _____.
- I feel ashamed when _____.[38]

While the child is being stripped of his parent-taught values in order to help him develop self-chosen values, he is at the same time bombarded with information. In drug prevention, the different categories of drugs, as well as their effects on the human being, are discussed. In death education, children are assigned to write their own epitaphs, write a suicide note, and—for first graders—to make a coffin for themselves out of a shoe box.[39] In sex education, as we have already discovered, homosexuality is presented as an alternative lifestyle, sexual techniques are discussed, including techniques for avoiding the consequences of sex—this method is 98 percent effective, while this one is only 88 percent safe. At no time is abstinence presented as an alternative lifestyle. In fact, at no time are any moral judgements passed.

We cannot help but wonder why they don't start a crime prevention class. As in the case of drug prevention and sex education, they can omit any moral judgments, and can simply discuss the different ways in which murders, burglaries, and shoplifting could be committed, as well as the various ways one could avoid detection. One does not need a high IQ to realize that amoral instruction in criminal issues would lead to an explosion in the crime rate. As we have seen, the effect of amoral instruction in sex has been an explosion in illegitimate pregnancies, abortions and sexually transmitted diseases.

Once again, however, statistics do not present the full story. The literature is simply overflowing with offensive cases of values clarification being applied in schools, as well as the heartbreaking stories of the children who had to take part in it. A so-called health class in a junior high school in Washington State required all the boys to say "vagina" in class and all the girls to say "penis." When one embarrassed girl was barely able to say it, the teacher "made her get up in front of the class and very loudly say it ten times."[40] Another class of children were told to write essays on "It's okay to try anything once," "A drug dealer is just a business person like anyone else," and "Do you think it's all right to lie, cheat, break laws once in a while, or only at certain times?"[41]

Joey, an 8-year-old boy, was part of a "problem solving" class in his school and was shown a film which depicted a young boy trying to kill himself by tying a rope around his neck. In the film, the boy talks about not being liked at school, being teased, and worrying about growing up. Joey's mother did not know about the program since the school curriculum merely stated that it was "social sciences." Two days after her son watched this video, she walked into his room and found him hanging by a rope from his bunk bed.[42]

Another student related the following:

> We had an English course in the ninth grade junior high whose title was "Death Education." In the manual, 73 out of 80 stories had to do with death, dying, killing, murder, suicide, and what you wanted on your tombstone. One girl, a ninth grader, blew her brains out after having written a note on her front door that said what she wanted on her tombstone.[43]

More of the Same

An occurrence that made the whole of America sit up straight was the report of the National Commission on Excellence in Education in April 1983. Referring to the collapse in standards at the secondary and college levels, the report stated: "Our Nation is at risk." The report warned that America would soon be engulfed by a "rising tide of mediocrity in elementary and secondary school."[44]

This report implicated that the new and improved curricula and teaching methods have ruined America's education. In order to reverse the decline, it would be logical to return to pre-1960s curricula, textbooks, and teaching methods. But the progressive educators of the 1990s had a new reform idea up their sleeves, *Outcomes Based Education* (OBE).

OBE did not just happen. It has been planned and worked out by humanist psychologists for years. The beginnings of OBE can be traced back to the 1948 meeting in Boston of the American Psychological Association Convention. At this meeting, a group of behavioral scientists decided to embark on a project of classifying the goals or outcomes of the education process since, as they said, "educational objectives provide the basis for building curricula and tests and represent the starting point for much of our educational research." The result of the scientists' deliberations has become known as Bloom's *Taxonomy of Educational Objectives*, a behavioral classification of outcomes produced by a new curriculum that does away with traditional subject matter and teaching methods. The central figure behind all this is behavioral scientist Benjamin S. Bloom of the University of Chicago.[45] A review of Bloom's book, *Human Characteristics and School Learning*, summarized what Bloom considered the aim of schools to be: "The school should work for equality of outcome and not for equality of opportunity, because the latter implies that there will be a range of outcomes due to a range of student's abilities, and this does not need to happen."[46]

This axiom of OBE has an oft-quoted corollary: all students can learn any subject matter if given enough time and teaching resources. To the humanists, the traditional system of education was fundamentally flawed in that some students received A's, some students received D's and F's, while most students received B's and C's. The flaw, as they perceive it, is that many of the children who received A's came from "advantaged" backgrounds, while many of the children who received C's, D's, and F's, came from "disadvantaged" backgrounds. In their worldview, the traditional system of education served to perpetuate the socioeconomic advantage or disadvantage that children brought with them to school. Thus, the traditional system of education is viewed as unfair, and in dire need of radical restructuring in order to level out the socioeconomic playing field.[47]

The fallaciousness of the idea that anyone can master calculus as well as Einstein if only given enough time should be as intuitively obvious as the absurdity of the idea that anyone can play basketball as well as Magic Johnson, or sing as well as Pavarotti, or sculpt as well as Michelangelo, if only he were given enough time and instruction. In the real world, achievement is a function of congenital ability and motivation. The traditional system of education recognized this truth. The children of high ability who worked hard got A's, the children of low ability and/or those who didn't work at all got F's, and everyone else fell somewhere in between. OBE advocates discount this truth and seek to replace it with the dangerous fantasy that achievement is solely a function of resources. If a child is achieving, it must be because of the child's privileged background. If a child isn't achieving, it is our collective fault because we haven't devoted enough resources.[48]

The problem is that the *only* way in which the goal of OBE— "an equality of outcome"—can be achieved, is by "dumbing down" classes. Many of the curricula being developed call for teachers to wait for all students to understand all aspects of a subject before moving on. Individuality is thus ignored, and creativity is stifled by group-think because a child cannot excel beyond his group. Equity is the goal—not excellence.[49] As Celano points out, these ideals are communist and socialist in nature:

> Rather than being encouraged to meet high standards and reap the rewards of individual excellence and achievement . . . [w]ork is done in groups, and grades are granted to groups. The kids who do no work get the same recognition and grade as those who did most of the work. There is no "dangerous" competition. There are no deadlines or standards to be met, save those of the lowest common denominator.[50]

OBE is clearly only a new name under which Dewey's, Rogers', and their followers' ideas live on. To quote Dr. Carl Rogers himself, "Change the name [of the reform policy] as fast as necessary to stay ahead of the critics."[51] In his book *Taxonomy of Educational Objec-*

tives, Benjamin Bloom states what the so-called outcomes should be:

> The curriculum may be thought of as a plan for changing students' behavior and as the actual set of learning experiences in which students, teachers, and materials interact to produce the change in students. . . . The careful observer of the classroom can see that the wise teacher as well as the psychological theorist use cognitive behavior and the achievement of cognitive goals to attain affective goals. . . . [A] large part of what we call "good teaching" is the teacher's ability to attain affective objectives through challenging the student's fixed beliefs.[52]

These outcomes indicate an intrusion into the personal and family lives of children, a facet that never seems to stop. As Luksik and Hoffecker point out, under the OBE model, schools will become "one-stop shopping for a child's every need." At the school of the future, children undergo at least twelve years of values clarification, in addition to other psychological games played by social workers.[53]

One of many criticisms that have been raised against OBE, is that there are no correct answers. William Glasser, one of OBE's promoters, wrote in his book *Schools Without Failure,* "We have to let students know there are no right answers, and we have to let them see that there are many alternatives to certainty and right answers."[54]

The track record of OBE, as was to be expected, has so far been very poor indeed. (1) Ballard High School in eastern Jefferson County, Kentucky, had a superb school record of academic excellence, until they introduced OBE. Tests showed that the failure rate was phenomenal and students were said to be "at risk." (2) The North Carolina Department of Public Instruction tested pilot OBE schools and compared them to non-OBE schools. For every subject, except U.S. history, the "OBE pilot sites as a whole scored anywhere from 1 to 11 percentile points below the state average." (3) Based on an objective test that has been used in the state for decades, Johnson City, New York, where OBE was used for twenty years, came last in reading, and nearly last in everything else.[55]

Sweden and Finland used to follow a similar system, but it has since been changed. Sweden's Minister of Education said of the system: "Swedish schools have diluted the quality of education by trying to do too much . . . [and have] neglected their basic function—educating children."[56] As Phyllis Schlafly, President of the Eagle Forum so rightly remarked, "OBE is converting the three R's to the three D's: Deliberately Dumbed Down."[57]

Finally, as if it were not enough to further compromise education in the United States by bringing in OBE, OBE-guru William Spady and his colleagues have, with the blessing of the U.S. government, taken this dog-and-pony show to South Africa. Billed as a helpful, post-apartheid humanitarian project, it was implemented under the name of *Curriculum 2005* with virtually no discussion. The South African government had been led to believe OBE was a proven technique that would vastly upgrade South African education.[58]

The Mental Hygiene Movement Joins the Educational Scene

As discussed, psychiatry, in the form of the Mental Hygiene Movement, expanded its activities beyond that of caretakers of the insane to caretakers of the general public.

In 1909, the National Committee for Mental Hygiene was formed. From its onset, the Committee sponsored studies that looked beyond a narrow defined notion of insanity. The first study, carried out in a Baltimore school in 1913, purported to show that 10 percent of the schoolchildren were in need of psychiatric assistance. Pilot programs were also begun at Sing Sing prison. The result of this research was that psychiatric departments were established in the juvenile courts and the prisons.[59]

The Mental Hygiene Movement, electing itself as an authority on the art of living and usurping the right to interfere with school and family for the public good, expanded rapidly. Children were an important target and from this movement evolved the child guidance movement, with the ultimate aim of *preventing* juvenile delinquency. Child guidance clinics, providing psychiatric intervention for pre-delinquent and problem children, sprang up overnight.[60]

Needless to say, the stated goal of preventing juvenile delinquency was never reached. As psychiatrist E. Fuller Torrey remarks, "Despite the proliferation of child guidance clinics and their popularity, no evidence was brought forth to suggest that the clinics prevented mental illness. The idea of preventing such illnesses, in fact, was largely ignored or forgotten during these years, and when it was raised at all it was done so with embarrassment."[61]

After failing to make headway with these children, the hygienists, instead of concluding that their ideas were wrong, deduced instead that *they hadn't intervened soon enough*.[62]

The Committee launched a parent education campaign in the 1920s, because it—as stated by Cohen and quoted in Wiseman's *Psychiatry: The Ultimate Betrayal*—believed parents to be too ignorant of child personality development to be trusted to raise children adequately. Unfortunately, this had the drawback of voluntary participation. Parents could not be forced to accept, listen to, or practice the good advice of the committee. Thus there remained only one alternative: the schools. As Ralph Truitt, the head of the Committee's Division of Child Guidance Clinics, stated in 1927, "the school should be the focus of our attack."

School failure was seen as the chief villain, leading to "feelings of inferiority," behavior problems like truancy or juvenile delinquency, withdrawal, an unsociable attitude, or a shut-up personality. The solution was clear. Eliminate the emphasis on academics. This, they reasoned, would rid the student of the stress of school failure. As psychiatrist and hygienist White wrote in 1927, education should be developed "as a scheme for assisting and guiding of the developing personality."

School discipline was another evil. Misbehavior in children was "not a sin, but a symptom." Cohen remarks, "Hygienists called upon the teacher to pay less attention to the child's overt behavior and more attention to understanding the motives, 'more or less unconscious,' underlying behavior, and over which the child had little control and for which the child could not be held responsible."[63]

Through large-scale marketing, the Committee's ideas filtered through to American decision-makers. In 1930 a White House Conference on Child Health and Protection was held, attracting some twelve hundred experts. A significant development at this conference was the involvement of an important group of psychologists who now wanted to pick up the mental hygiene banner. *All* were from Teachers College. The year 1930 thus marked the marriage of the purposes of the Progressive Education Association and the National Committee for Mental Hygiene.[64] Hand in hand, psychology and psychiatry now worked together to bring about the decay of morality and the collapse of education that were to follow a few decades later.

In 1948, as previously mentioned, the World Federation for Mental Health was formed, cofounded by Rees and Chisholm. In 1950, the National Committee for Mental Hygiene faded, combining with several organizations to become the National Association for Mental Health. As the Mental Hygiene Movement expanded, its ideas infiltrated American life and education, and slowly but surely beyond the borders of the United States.

In 1952, the first DSM was published, listing 112 "mental disorders." By 1994, the list had grown to 374. In the DSM, psychiatry had found an excuse for its inability to prevent or solve the problems of adults and children. At the same time, parents and teachers were relieved of the guilt feelings that had been brought about by behaviorism. The question, "Where did we go wrong?" was increasingly replaced by the idea that nobody could be held accountable for the child's problems, because the child was suffering from an incurable disease.

Psychiatry reached a further important milestone in 1962. By reporting alarming statistics of "mental illness" within society—without providing any proof of these—psychiatrists convinced governors attending a governor's conference in 1962 to pass resolutions calling on all states to fund psychiatric programs.[65]

Yet by far the most important victory for psychiatry and psychology came in 1965 with the passage of the Elementary and Secondary Education Act (ESEA). The ESEA allocated massive federal funds and opened the school doors to a flood of psychiatrists, psychologists, psychiatric programs, and psychological testing that continues to this day. The number of educational psychologists in the United States increased from 455 in 1969 to 16,146 in 1992.[66] As of 1994, child psychiatrists, psychologists, counselors, and special educators in and around the U.S. public schools nearly outnumbered teachers.[67] Now there were a great many to follow in the footsteps of Carl Rogers, who could, in his words, "choose to use [their] . . . knowledge to enslave people in ways never dreamed of before, depersonalizing them, controlling them by means so carefully selected that they will perhaps never be aware of their loss of personhood."[68]

Notes

1. Mead, M., "Thinking ahead: Why is education so obsolete?" *Harvard Business Review* 36, November-December 1958.

2. Adams, C., "OBE: A crash course in dumbing down," website.

3. Rohlen, T. P., *Japan's High Schools* (Berkeley: University of California Press, 1983).

4. Honig, B., *Last Chance for Our Children* (New York: Addison-Wesley Publishing, Inc., 1987), 30.

5. Sowell, T., *Inside American Education* (Englewood Cliffs: Julian Messner, 1993), 12.

6. Cohen, S., "The Mental Hygiene Movement, the development of personality and the school: The medicalization of American education," *History of Education Quarterly*, Summer 1983, 129, cited in Wiseman, *Psychiatry: The Ultimate Betrayal* (Los Angeles: Freedom Publishing, 1995), 267.

7. Lionni, P., & Klass, L. J., *The Leipzig Connection: The Systematic Destruction of American Education* (Portland: Oregon: Heron Books, 1980), 42.

8. Wiseman, *Psychiatry: The Ultimate Betrayal*, 259.

9. Ibid., 260-261.

10. Lionni & Klass, *The Leipzig Connection*.

11. Idomir, L. S., *The Tangled Web. Humanism: Enrichment or Enslavement?* (Conway: Alert, 1989), 4.

12. Van Wyk, J. H., *Strominge in die Opvoedingsteorie* (Butterworth), 36-37.

13. Idomir, *The Tangled Web*, 20.

14. breakpoint.org/scripts/60624.htm, website.

15. Eakman, B. K., *Cloning of the American Mind: Eradicating Morality through Education* (Lafayette: Huntington House Publishers, 1998), 120.

16. Ibid.

17. Wiseman, *Psychiatry: The Ultimate Betrayal*, 262-264.

18. *Newsweek*, 1976, cited in J. P. Dworetzky, *Introduction to Child Development* (St. Paul, Minnesota: West Publishing Co., 1981), 447-448.

19. Blumenfeld, S. L., *N.E.A.: Trojan Horse in American Education* (Boise, Idaho: The Paradigm Company, 1984).

20. Ibid.

21. Nelson-Jones, R., *The Theory and Practice of Counselling Psychology* (London: Holt, Pinehart and Winston, 1982), 16-17.

22. Engler, B., *Personality Theories: An Introduction* (Boston: Houghton Mifflin Company, 1979), 302.

23. Idomir, *The Tangled Web*, 21.

24. Ibid.

25. Rogers, C., *Freedom to Learn for the 80's* (Columbus, Ohio: Charles E. Merrill Publishing Co., 1983), 3.

26. Rogers, C., & Stevens, B., (eds.), *Person to Person: The Problem of Being Human* (Lafayette: Real People Press, 1967), 58-61, cited in R. F. Biehler, *Psychology Applied to Teaching* (3rd ed.), (Boston: Houghton Mifflin Company, 1978), 341.

27. Rogers, *Freedom to Learn for the 80's*, 136-137.

28. Sowell, T., *Inside American Education* (Englewood Cliffs: Julian Messner, 1993), 90.

29. Rogers, *Freedom to Learn for the 80's*, 288.

30. Sowell, *Inside American Education*, 90.

31. Ibid., 90-91.

32. Ibid., 91-92.

33. Ibid., 5.

34. Eakman, *Cloning of the American Mind*, 21.

35. Ibid., 94.

36. Robinson, J., *Attack on the Family* (Tyndale Press, 1982), 90, cited in J. M. Wallis, *The Disaster Road* (Bullsbrook: Veritas Publishing Company Pty. Ltd., 1986), 46.

37. Sowell, *Inside American Education*, 45.

38. Ibid., 46.

39. Ibid., 37.

40. Ibid., 39.

41. "Meddling with minds," *Education: Psychiatry's Ruin* (Los Angeles: CCHR, 1995), 16-21.

42. Ibid.

43. Ibid.

44. Kantrowitz, B., et al., "A nation still at risk," *Newsweek*, 19 April 1993, 46-49.

45. "Questions answered on: OBE," website.

46. *International Review of Education* (New York: McGraw Hill, 1976), 139, cited in Wallis, *The Disaster Road*, 40.

47. "OBE: What is it? Where did it come from?" Part 5, 1996-1997, *Gateway Citizens for Educational Reform.*

48. Ibid.

49. Adams, "OBE: A crash course in dumbing down."

50. Celano, P. J., "Outcome Based Education," 1996, website.

51. Ibid.

52. Ibid.

53. Luksik, P. & Hoffecker, P. H., *Outcome-Based Education: The State's Assault on Our Children's Values* (Lafayette, Louisiana: Huntington House Publishers, 1995), cited in "Reviews: The educational Trojan Horse known as Outcome-Based Education comes under scrutiny by these authors," website.

54. Celano, "Outcome Based Education."

55. "Questions answered on: OBE."

56. *Wall Street Journal,* 7 April 1992.

57. Schlafly, P., "What's wrong with Outcomes Based Education?" *The Phyllis Schlafly Report,* May 1993, 4.

58. Eakman, *Cloning of the American Mind,* 344.

59. Castel, R. et al., *The Psychiatric Society,* translated by A. Goldhammer, (Chicago: University of Illinois Press, 1982), 28, cited in Wiseman, *Psychiatry: The Ultimate Betrayal,* 72.

60. Wiseman, *Psychiatry: The Ultimate Betrayal,* 73, 75, 267.

61. Torrey, E. F., *Nowhere to Go* (New York: Harper and Row, 1988), 50, cited in Wiseman, *Psychiatry: The Ultimate Betrayal,* 76.

62. Cohen, "The Mental Hygiene Movement," 124, cited in Wiseman, *Psychiatry: The Ultimate Betrayal,* 267.

63. Cohen, "The Mental Hygiene Movement," 124-145, cited in Wiseman, *Psychiatry: The Ultimate Betrayal,* 267-268.

64. Wiseman, *Psychiatry: The Ultimate Betrayal,* 269.

65. "The beginning of the end," *Education: Psychiatry's Ruin* (Los Angeles: CCHR, 1995), 4-11.

66. Fagan, T. K., "NASP as a force for improving school psychology: What have been its accomplishments?" Annual convention, National Association of School Psychologists, Washington, D.C., 1993, cited in "The beginning of the end," *Education: Psychiatry's Ruin.*

67. "The beginning of the end," *Education: Psychiatry's Ruin.*

68. Pacard, V., *The People Shapers* (New York: Bantam Books, Inc., 1979), inside leaf page, cited in "Rogerian therapy destroys religious orders," *Psychiatry Destroying Religion* (Los Angeles: CCHR, 1997), 22-23.

10.

The "Heart" of Psychology and Psychiatry

A one-third-page newspaper advertisement on Adolescent Behavioral Health sponsored by a large hospital shows a teenage boy with his arm around his girlfriend. They are dressed in punk outfits. The ad says, "Young people frequently choose hairstyles and clothing to express healthy adolescent rebellion. But how is one to tell whether his teenager's behavior is OK or self-destructive?" The answer is obvious: "The professionals at the Behavioral Health System ... are here to assist you in answering this crucial question.... We will help you.... Call someone you can trust."[1]

According to the advertisement, professionals are able to make a clear distinction between healthy adolescent rebellion and self-destructive adolescent behavior. Besides the fact that a parent should run a million miles away from any professional claiming rebellious behavior to be healthy, the advertisement strengthens a false belief in the capabilities of psychology and its medical equal. In the words of Schrag and Divoky, the experts have built a mystical aura around them, using modern techniques, screens and tests to diagnose and treat children. They pretend to be capable of seeing things in the child that the layman can never see.[2] As shown in the advertisement above, they want us to believe them capable of telling the difference between healthy adolescent rebellion and self-destructive adolescent behavior. What parents are not aware of is that when such distinctions are made, they are not based on knowledge or scientific processes of any kind, but merely on fabrication based on invented criteria. And, as self-destructive adolescent behavior has a financial incentive far greater than healthy rebellious behavior, in all probability the former is what the diagnosis will be.

As stated above, to a person who has a hammer in his hand, everything looks like a nail. Over the past years, we have become acquainted with many of the hammers used by psychiatry and its cohorts. There is, for example, one expert who calls his hammer "Tourette's syndrome." (This problem and the way it relates to ADHD will be discussed below.) For nearly five consecutive years, at an average rate of two per week, we have had the opportunity to speak to parents whose children have been through the consulting rooms of this person. Whenever his name is mentioned, our immediate reaction—which has become automatic by now—is: "Oh, so your child has Tourette's syndrome?" to which the parent would usually react with a surprised, "Oh, how do you know?" The worst is that these children who often have to live with this stigma for the rest of their lives seldom show the usual symptoms that are associated with "Tourette's syndrome," (i.e. the so-called motor or verbal tics.)

One cannot but feel doubtful when left with the impression that every person who enters the consultation rooms of a professional seems to suffer from the same disease. When one further observes that there seem to be several professionals who appear to have his own individual hammer that he applies to every person who enters his consulting rooms, one's suspicions become overwhelming. Such subjective observations on the unscientific character of psychological and psychiatric—and related—diagnostic practices have been confirmed by numerous studies.

One study examined the extent to which professionals were able to differentiate so-called "learning-disabled" (LD) students from "ordinary" low achievers by examining scores on psychometric measures. Subjects were 65 school psychologists, 38 special education teachers, and a naive group of 21 university students enrolled in programs unrelated to education or psychology. Provided with forms containing information on 41 test or subtest scores (including the WISC-R IQ test) of nine school-identified LD students and nine non-LD students, judges were instructed to indicate which students they believed were learning disabled and which were non-learning disabled.[3]

The results of this experiment demonstrate quite clearly why some commentators have been led to label the current practices a "diagnostic scandal."[4] The school psychologists and special education teachers were able to differentiate between LD students and low achievers with only 50 percent accuracy. The naive judges, who had never had more than an introductory course in education or psychology, evidenced a 75 percent hit rate.[5]

Another experiment at Stanford University showed how easily the experts can be fooled. D.L. Rosenhan, professor of psychology and law at Stanford University, had eight "perfectly sane people" (Rosenhan himself, one graduate student, three psychologists, a pediatrician, a psychiatrist, and a homemaker)[6] admitted to twelve different mental hospitals. The attending psychiatrists were told that these "patients" were hearing voices:

> Otherwise, these normal people . . . gave completely truthful histories to the psychiatrists. They were all diagnosed as "schizophrenic," except one who was diagnosed as "manic-depressive." Once admitted, they acted perfectly normally; yet were held for 7 to 52 days (the average was 19) and were given over 2,100 pills total. The true patients on the wards often recognized them as pseudopatients but the staff never did. Once labeled, the staff's perception of them was apparently so profoundly colored that normal behavior was seen as part of the psychosis.
>
> In an even more damning postscript to the experiment, Rosenhan told one hospital what he had done. He then told them that he would try to gain admission for another pseudopatient there within the next 3 months. Ever watchful for the pseudopatient who was never sent, the staff labeled 41 of the next 193 admissions as suspected pseudopatients; over half of these were so labeled by a psychiatrist. The experimenter concluded: "Any diagnostic process that lends itself so readily to massive errors of this sort cannot be very reliable."[7]

The Proof of the Pudding

Psychology and psychiatry could easily have been forgiven these diagnostic flaws if they had been able to effect positive changes in the conditions of their patients. After all, the proof of the pudding is in the eating. The unpleasant truth, however, is that these disciplines are ineffective in changing thought and behavior patterns. As the outspoken Schrag and Divoky remarked, "The power of [psychological and psychiatric] systems does not depend on results any more than did the power of the witch doctor . . . the larger the armamentarium of routines, the greater the mystification. What paint and feathers and mumbo-jumbo did for the shaman, screens, computers and syndromes can do for the diagnostician."[8]

In 1952, a study by Eysenck demonstrated that recovery from neuroses is unrelated to whether a patient receives *any* form of psychotherapy. Some researchers have challenged Eysenck's conclusions and have stated that there is general agreement that psychotherapy is at least better than no therapy.[9]

Further research tended to show the opposite. To prove his point, Eysenck did a second study in 1965, and according to Martin Gross, this study was:

> a more extensive survey of published studies, with still more damaging results for psychotherapy. He now claims that psychotherapy is a general failure by the very nature of its being unessential to the patient's recovery. "We have found that neurotic disorders tend to be self-limiting, that psychoanalysis is no more successful than any other method, and that in fact all methods of psychotherapy fail to improve on the recovery rate obtained through ordinary life-experiences and nonspecific treatment."[10]

Eysenck's research was an explosive revelation that psychotherapy is a failure and absolutely inessential. Not surprisingly, many psychologists hotly disputed his conclusions. As a result, Eysenck's work has been reexamined. A review of his research by Truax and Carkhuff claims to validate his conclusions. In fact, they even go further when they state, "The evidence now available suggests that, on the average, psychotherapy may be harmful as often as helpful, with an average effect comparable to receiving no help."[11]

Another damning review of 42 studies comparing the effectiveness of professional therapists with those of little training, found that the trained counselors were significantly more effective in only one of the studies. In the majority, the professionals and paraprofessionals were equally effective and in twelve of the reports the less trained counselors came out ahead.[12]

Equally damaging to psychology's claims is the Cambridge-Somerville Youth Study, reported in 1978 in *American Psychologist*. This thirty year study revealed that men, who had received an average of five years of psychotherapy as boys, were in worse shape, in view of alcoholism, criminal behavior, and mental disorders, than those who had not undergone psychotherapy.[13]

Over the past few years we have tried to keep abreast of the work of several Christian psychologists and pastoral psychologists, believing that they might be better equipped to help people in need.

Our conclusion is that the differences between Christian and pastoral psychologists and secular psychologists are so minuscule that one needs a magnifying glass to see them. There may be exceptions, but so far we have not been able to come across one who attaches more value to the Bible than to the DSM. For example, when a person swears, he is viewed as sinful, but when he swears continually he supposedly suffers from "Tourette's syndrome." A person who steals is a thief, but the one who steals persistently suffers from kleptomania. A child who ignores his parent's instructions is disobedient, but those who are habitually disobedient suffer from ADHD. Lastly, their advice on child rearing is seldom different from the advice found in child education books authored by behaviorists.

The reason for the small distinction between Christian and pastoral psychology and secular psychology can perhaps be found in the following admission, made by a psychologist:

> Because psychologists have spent up to nine years studying psychology in school and are pressed to spend much of their reading time in their field in order to stay current, it is inevitable that we develop a certain "mind-set." The all-too-common but disastrous result is that we tend to look at Scripture through the eyeglasses of psychology when the critical need is to look at psychology through the glasses of Scripture.[14]

Indeed, if one looks at psychology through the glasses of Scripture, the term Christian or pastoral psychology becomes a total anomaly. One cannot serve both God and psychology. The same applies to psychiatry. As Röder et al. remarked, "Any religion . . . which teaches the existence of God or the immortality of the soul will recognize psychiatry for what it is and realize that any 'conciliation' will come at their peril."[15] One has to make a choice—and if you find it difficult to accept this point of view, maybe the following bit of incriminating evidence will help you to reach a verdict.

The Hidden Agendas of the "Experts"

The failures in consulting rooms seem minuscule compared to the failures of our two cousins in the classrooms. As Sowell implies, there seems to be a direct connection between the number of school psychologists and mental health workers and the increase in illiteracy, youth violence, teenage promiscuity, and teen suicide:

Barely more than half the people employed at the New York
City Board of Education are teachers ... Moreover, one-
third of the money that trickles down the school goes for
psychologists and counselors alone ... What has gotten better in American schools after we have flooded them with
psychologists, counselors, "facilitators" and the
like? ... Academic performance certainly hasn't improved.
We have yet to see test scores as high as they were 30 years
ago. Maybe students are happier, healthier or something. But
statistics on cheating, theft, vandalism, violent crime, venereal disease and teenage suicide all say no.[16]

Contrary to what most people believe, the chaos in schools has
not been the result of stupid thinking, but of careful and continuous
planning of humanist psychologists and psychiatrists. Unfortunately,
if one considers the actions and pronouncements that have ema-
nated from their ranks over the past few decades, one cannot but
conclude that it has never been one of their aims to provide a proper
education to children. As U.S. circuit court judge Patrick J. Madden
wrote, "[these] educational theorists [are] seemingly ... more concerned with social engineering than with [the] education ... of our
children."[17] The deeper one delves into the motives of these theorists, the more it becomes clear that they have everything but literacy and proficiency on their agendas. Their agendas rather seem
to be to create chaos.

To fully understand why anybody would deliberately want the
educational system to collapse, one must begin with the "Father of
Progressive Education," John Dewey. Dewey, like his followers, was
a "humanist"—a term synonymous with atheist.

Simply stated, the idea of humanism is to reform society. As Dr.
Cuddy explains, "If there is no god to Whom to pray, and if man
simply evolved, he must depend solely upon himself to solve the
world's problems."[18] It appears that, for humanists, this means that
a new social world order must replace patriotism and nationalism,
a new world religion must replace Christianity and Judaism, and
amorality must replace biblical and traditional values. The public
schools, it seems, play a central role in achieving this humanist ideal.
As Dr. Just remarked, "Everyone behind the New Education, the
'Relevant-Creative-Do-It-Yourself Education' talks of creating a new
society through the children."[19]

Dewey, who coauthored and cosigned the atheist *Humanist
Manifesto I,* believed that public schools should "take active part in

determining the social order of the future."[20] He and his progressive followers envisioned a school system of social engineering, changing attitudes, and changing values, and therefore they commandeered teachers to align themselves as forces of social change and economic control.[21] In the May 1949 issue of *Progressive Educator* magazine, Kenneth Benne wrote, "Teachers and school administrators should come to see themselves as social engineers. They must equip themselves as change agents."[22]

According to Morris Storer's book, *Humanist Ethics,* these "change agents" are readily available. He asserts that "a large majority of the educators of American colleges and universities are predominantly humanists, and a majority of teachers who go out from their studies in colleges to responsibilities in primary and secondary schools are basically humanist, no matter that many maintain nominal attachment to church or synagogue for personal and social or practical reasons."[23] Even prior to the first *Humanist Manifesto,* Charles Potter came to the same conclusion. In his book *Humanism: A New Religion,* published in 1930, he wrote:

> Education is thus a most powerful ally of humanism, and every American public school is a school of humanism. What can the theistic Sunday schools, meeting for an hour a week, and teaching only a fraction of the children, do to stem the tide of a five-day program of humanistic teaching?[24]

By the time when Dewey was cowriting the first *Humanist Manifesto,* another psychologist and revolutionary Marxist, Erich Fromm, arrived on the scene. Fromm wrote, among other books, *The Dogma of Christ and Other Essays on Religion, Psychology, and Care.* Apart from trashing Jesus, the book developed a concept of the modern man-ideal: a political-psychological revolutionary figure. To be called "revolutionary" was a compliment. "The revolutionary," wrote Fromm, "is the man who has emancipated himself from the ties of blood and soil, from his mother and father, from special loyalties to state, class, race, party, or religion. The Revolutionary character is a Humanist." As Eakman tells us, Fromm was also the first to impose the idea upon psychologists and psychiatrists to become revolutionary characters. Brock Chisholm, Ewen Cameron and J. R. Rees, who followed Fromm, in reality only modernized Fromm's verbiage for the World War II and postwar generations, where it eventually took hold in earnest in the form of the Mental Hygiene Movement.[25]

Capitalizing on the cumulative efforts of Thorndike, Dewey, Freud, Fromm, and others, states Eakman:

> the 1960s ensured that an entire generation was brought up with the idea that rebellion against anything even remotely perceived as being repressive was both mentally healthy and politically necessary and that a person's feelings had priority over logic and thought. This constituted a time bomb, waiting for the right fuse. That fuse . . . was drugs. Meanwhile, the forces known as "social decomposition," including divorce, illegitimacy, sexual perversion, disrespect for and abuse of the elderly, and "sick" entertainment are slowly overtaking the positive social forces and "civilizing influences."[26]

While society was crumbling, the role of teachers as change agents of humanism were shifting more and more from the imparting of knowledge, the cultivation of scholarship, and of the intellect, to the achieving of the humanistic ideal—the transformation of society.[27] This was not only the case in the United States, but throughout the Western world. In 1993, Manuela Friehofer of Zurich, Switzerland, described the detour the Swiss education has taken—from its former incarnation as perhaps the finest in the world, to its current emotion-laden atmosphere which "breaks every boundary of decency and human dignity":

> For the past 20 years our association has observed with increasing alarm the systematic dismantling, not just of the Swiss education system, but also of social and political structures too. . . . [A] political battle is being fought in our schools, and the victims are, of course, the pupils.

> Teachers, who use traditional methods, are branded as child murderers, prison wardens and sadists. We are continually told that scientifically tried and tested teaching methods damage and dull a child's development. . . . "[R]eformers" have managed to brainwash parents and teachers with the help of the media. Pupils are said to be imprisoned at school, the work the children do to resemble that of idiots in a lunatic asylum. These people have already succeeded in pushing through the changes: . . . Pupils are encouraged to live out and to experience their "true" feelings such as anger, aggression, and hate. "Project week" and "discovery learning" result in children spending more time in the woods and on walks than in the classroom. It is not surprising that when

children do have to concentrate on work, they are just not able to. An atmosphere of learning is no longer created, in fact it is despised. . . .

Hand in hand with these reforms are the changes being realized in the teachers' training institutions. Left-wing radicals in universities and . . . colleges systematically subject their students to a kind of training that breaks every boundary of decency and human dignity. One of the hair-raising examples experienced by primary school teachers can be observed in a psychology lesson whose title was "The Anal Phase." A questionnaire contained, amongst others, the following bizarre questions:

• What does your excrement and urine smell like?
• Are you disturbed by your own noises whilst going to the toilet?
• How do you behave on the toilet at home?
• Do you enjoy spending some time on the toilet?
• How do you clean yourself and how do you clean the toilet?
• How do you cope with menstruation?[28]

Beverly Eakman did an extensive study on this topic. According to Eakman, the social transformation is being engineered not by one but by two equally unethical cadres of behavioral scientists of the Mental Hygiene Movement—one being eugenic psychologists/psychiatrists and evolutionary psychologists, and the other being essentially professional Marxist agitators.[29]

The word *eugenics* was coined by Francis Galton, a half-cousin of Charles Darwin. Galton was by no means satisfied to let evolution take its course freely, and thus extended Darwin's theory of natural selection into a concept of deliberate social intervention. The Nazis took this idea to extremes by murdering 275,000 mental patients from 1939 to 1945, and by exterminating millions of Jews.[30]

As the Nazis did, the eugenicists and evolutionary psychologists believe that they can create a superior race. They are thus interested in removing "defectives" and "cleaning up the gene pool,"[31] in order to "minimize the damage to evolution."[32] Linda Erlenmeyer-Kimling, former president of the American Eugenics Society-cum-Society for the Study of Social Biology, outlined their purpose:

The essence of evolution is natural selection; the essence of eugenics is the replacement of "natural" selection by conscious, premeditated or artificial selection in the hope of speeding up the evolution of "desirable" characteristics and the elimination of "undesirable" ones.[33]

The "defectives" who are polluting the gene pool and have to be weeded out are the poor, illiterate, mentally handicapped, and mentally disturbed,[34] as well as people holding unacceptable beliefs. *They* are seen as "defective" as well. If you thus believe in a spiritual dimension or moral codes (referred to as *absolutism* by detractors), you are defective, or mentally ill.[35] "There is a common, close association between religion and psychotic disorders," psychiatrist Eli S. Chesen stated in his book *Religion May Be Hazardous to Your Health.*[36] To "clean up the gene pool," man must thus be freed from his concept of right and wrong.

Since Linda Erlenmeyer-Kimling determined that ADHD was a behavioral marker for so-called schizophrenia, children with ADHD are therefore also viewed as defectives. She subsequently urged for mass screening programs so that intervention and, if possible, prevention could be made in the form of *population control.* The easiest place for such mass screening to be done was in the classroom. In the words of Erlenmeyer-Kimling, "compulsory education is of service to eugenics."[37]

From what we could gather, abortion is only one way of weeding out life's defectives. If they could have their way, they would have compulsory sterilization programs. One suggestion is that all females should have a drug administered at puberty in the form of a time capsule implanted under the skin so that it would produce long-term sterility reversible only through the administration of another drug. Prospective parents would have to demonstrate their "genetic superiority," while unlicensed babies would immediately have to be relinquished by their mothers and be placed in government custody. A presupposition for the effectiveness of such a plan is the presumption that "most pregnant women would rather seek an abortion than suffer the substantial emotional pain of relinquishing their baby with the prospect of never seeing it again."[38]

At this point, eugenicists began working more closely with pharmacologists, and a whole new field of psychopharmacology opened up, eventually giving us Valium, Prozac, Zoloft, and other mood-enhancers, "some of which happen to have, as a potent side effect, the reduction of sexual drive and even sexual dysfunction."[39]

What is interesting about this drama, however, is that the eugenicists' mission, to improve the racial stock, was to go astray through the more aggressive efforts of the Marxist Left. These psychologists were not interested in "cleaning up the gene pool," but in instigating chaos, and to accomplish that required as much illegitimacy, crime, single parenthood, consumer debt, and social isolation as possible. So, if you are puzzled as to why American society and other societies appear to be pushing abortion rights at the same time it is promoting illegitimacy through graphic, early sex education, and through financial incentives favoring cohabiting partners, says Eakman, the answer is that you have two separate factions at work.[40]

Yet, as the endgames of these factions are not so far apart—freedom from concepts about right and wrong and an economy based on what they call today free-market socialism—they joined hands in the 1970s.[41] If one uses as example the practice of values clarification, one can clearly see how the same practice has come to serve the selfish and atheistic ideals of both factions.

What makes values clarification so successful in the hands of a change agent is its principal ingredient—the manner in which students are led to believe they are choosing their own values, when in fact, they are being led to a predetermined conclusion. This predetermined conclusion is that they (our children) are autonomous ("autonomy" means shedding the restrictions and authority of parental and religious requirements) and can decide for themselves what is right and wrong.[42] *Autonomy* is important for the eugenicists and evolutionary psychologists, as it "cures" our children from a severe "mental illness"—believing in God and living by moral codes.

The Kinsey studies, financed by the Rockefeller Foundation in the mid-twentieth century, cast a glance at a world without such moral restraints:

> In cases involving molestation of young girls by adult men, Kinsey held that the real damage was done by cultural conditioning. The child is "constantly warned" by adults, parents, and teachers against strange men, and as a result they are "emotionally upset or frightened by their contacts with adults." . . . The real offender is not the adult child molester but the inhibiting parent and society with their moral "thou shalt nots."[43]

If one looks around, it becomes clear that we are not far from the anarchistic paradise Alfred C. Kinsey portrayed in his studies. As Eakman points out, in recent years:

the public has become more amused than disgusted by the increasingly graphical and detailed sexual misadventures reported about our nation's leaders, film stars, and other public figures. Pedophiles and pornographers argue their cases on talk shows, personal ads in mainstream magazines are replete with sexual offers. Lesbian groups distribute fliers to eight-year-olds on an elementary campus. Condoms are made to look cutesy in TV commercials aimed at the younger set and are served up like greeting cards at the dorm rooms of entering college freshmen.[44]

As already indicated, values clarification is also of service to the Marxist Left. If the schools teach dependence on one's self (autonomy), H. J. Blackham, a founder of the International Humanist Ethic Union, stated in the September-October 1981 issue of *The Humanist,* "they are more revolutionary than any conspiracy to overthrow the government . . . [and] sustained pressure from this quarter [meaning everyone pressing for their own interest] moves a society . . . in the direction of world order.[45]

Besides nationalism and Christianity, parents and families are the obstacles in the way of these humanistic ideals. In a campaign against parents and families, Dr. Reginald Lourie announced to the British Humanist Association in the document "Marriage and Family":

> The Humanist view is that marriage is a human institution . . . in no way sacred and immutable. Some opponents of Humanism have accused us of wishing to overthrow the Traditional Christian Family. They are right. That is exactly what we intend to do.[46]

And the way in which they intend to overthrow the traditional Christian family is by brainwashing our children in the classroom with psychological exercises such as values clarification—the values clarified being authoritarian and Judeo-Christian ones. As Paul Blanchard boasted in 1976 in *The Humanist:*

> I think the most important factor moving us toward a secular society has been the education factor. Our schools may not teach Johnny to read properly but the fact that Johnny is in school until he is 16 tends to lead toward the elimination of religious superstition. The average American child now acquires a high school education, and this militates against Adam and Eve and all the other myths of alleged

history.[47]

In 1983, writing for the January-February issue of *The Humanist*, John Dunphy echoed Blanchard's optimism:

> I am convinced that the battle for humankind's future will be waged and won in the public school classrooms by teachers who correctly perceive their role as proselytizers of a new faith . . . [The war is] between the rotting corpse of Christianity . . . and the future faith of humanism . . . [and] humanism will emerge triumphant.[48]

Reflecting on the chaos in schools, Samuel Blumenfeld stated in 1984, "It's time the American [and Australian, and European, and South African] consumer knew the extent of the fraud which is victimizing millions of children each year. A consumer can sue a private company for shoddy goods and misrepresentation . . . But a student whose life has been ruined by educational malpractice in a public school has no recourse to the law. The educators are accountable to no one but themselves." Then he added—and we cannot agree more—"It's time the fraud was stopped. It's time for people to rise and throw off a tyranny that can only get worse if nothing is done. There is a time to stand up and be counted. That time is *now* (our italics)."[49]

It is also time for parents to turn their backs on the ridiculous and outlandish advice of experts on child rearing. One has to be blind not to see that their foolproof methods are not foolproof at all. In fact, their advice has caused our children to be violent, rebellious, selfish, defiant, promiscuous, and unhappy. There is nothing wrong with our children. They do not have ADHD, ODD, and CD. There is only something wrong with the expert advice we, their parents, have so ignorantly followed. Knowing the truth, however, will enable us to make a choice—a choice between the poisonous ideas of psychology and psychiatry and the time-honored traditions of childcare, which have harvested generations of decent and respectable citizens. The time to make that choice is *now!*

Notes

1. *Rocky Mountain News*, 30 January 1992, 51, cited in E. Bulkley, *Why Christians Can't Trust Psychology* (Eugene, Oregon: Harvest House Publishers, 1993), 72.

2. Schrag, P., & Divoky, D., *The Myth of the Hyperactive Child and Other Means of Child Control* (Middlesex: Penguin Books, 1975).

3. Epps, S., Ysseldyke, J. E., & McGue, M., "I know one when I see one: Differentiating LD and non LD-students," *Learning Disability Quarterly*, vol. 7, 1984, 89-101.

4. Scriven, M., "Comments on Gene Class," Paper presented at the Wingspread National Invitational Conference on Public Policy and the Special Education Task of the 1980s, cited in D. P. Hallahan, J. Kauffman & J. Lloyd, *Introduction to Learning Disabilities* (Englewood Cliffs, NJ: Prentice Hall, 1985), 298.

5. Ysseldyke, J. E., & Algozzine, B., "LD or not LD: That's not the question!" *Journal of Learning Disabilities*, vol. 16(1), 1983, 26-27.

6. Striano, J., *How to Find a Good Psychotherapist: A Consumer Guide* (Santa Barbara, CA: Professional Press, 1987), 79, cited in Bulkley, *Why Christians Can't Trust Psychology*, 75.

7. Torrey, E. F., *The Death of Psychiatry* (Radnor, PA: Little, Brown and Company, 1974), 47.

8. Schrag & Divoky, *The Myth of the Hyperactive Child.*

9. Bulkley, *Why Christians Can't Trust Psychology*, 73.

10. Gross, M. L., *The Psychological Society* (New York: Random House, 1978), 23, cited in Bulkley, *Why Christians Can't Trust Psychology*, 73.

11. Gross, *The Psychological Society*, 40, cited in Bulkley, *Why Christians Can't Trust Psychology*, 73.

12. Durlak, J. A., "Comparative effectiveness of paraprofessionals and professional helpers," *Psychological Bulletin*, 86, 1979, 88-89, cited in B. Wiseman, *Psychiatry: The Ultimate Betrayal* (Los Angeles: Freedom Publishing, 1995), 40.

13. Bobgan, M., & Bobgan, D., *Psychoheresy* (Santa Barbara, CA: EastGate Publishers, 1987), cited in Bulkley, *Why Christians Can't Trust Psychology*, 74.

14. Crabb, L. J., Jr., *Basic Principles of Biblical Counseling* (Grand Rapids: Zondervan Publishing House, 1977), 48.

15. Röder, T., Kubillus, V., & Burwell, A., *Psychiatrists: The Men Behind Hitler* (Los Angeles: Freedom Publishing, 1994), 321.

16. Sowell, T., "There's no problem so big that we can't make it worse," *Rocky Mountain News*, 20 February 1992, 49.

17. "Questions answered on: OBE," website.

18. Cuddy, D. L., "Secular humanism in our schools," *The Union Leader (Manchester Edition)*, 21 May 1985, cited in J. M. Wallis, *The Disaster Road* (Bullsbrook: Veritas Publishing Company Pty. Ltd., 1986), 58.

19. Wallis, *The Disaster Road*, 24.

20. Dewey, J., 1896, cited in G. Allen, "New education," *American Opinion*, May 1971, 4.

21. Eakman, B. K., *Cloning of the American Mind: Eradicating Morality through Education* (Lafayette: Huntington House Publishers, 1998), 121.

22. Cuddy, D. L., *20 Years of Federal Change Agentry*, 1.

23. Cuddy, D. L., "Secular humanism in our schools," cited in Wallis, *The Disaster Road*, 53.

24. Ibid.

25. Eakman, *Cloning of the American Mind*, 149-150.

26. Ibid., 233.

27. Wallis, *The Disaster Road*, 24.

28. Friehofer, M., "The death of education," *The Salisbury Review*, September 1993, cited in Eakman, *Cloning of the American Mind*, 238-239.

29. Eakman, B. K., "The worldwide threat of behavioral science in education," Speech delivered on 1 March 1999.

30. Wiseman, *Psychiatry: The Ultimate Betrayal*, 61-66.

31. Eakman, "The worldwide threat of behavioral science in education."

32. Eakman, *Cloning of the American Mind*, 176.

33. Ibid.

34. Ibid., 174.

35. Eakman, "The worldwide threat of behavioral science in education."

36. Chesen, E. I., *Religion May Be Hazardous to Your Health*, cited in Röder, Kubillus & Burwell, *Psychiatrists: The Men Behind Hitler*, 320.

37. Eakman, *Cloning of the American Mind*, 174.

38. Heer, D. M., *Social Biology*, vol. 2(1), 1975, cited in Eakman, *Cloning of the American Mind*, 180.

39. Eakman, *Cloning of the American Mind*, 181.

40. Eakman, "The worldwide threat of behavioral science in education."

41. Ibid.

42. *Alert*, June 1985, 3, cited in Wallis, *The Disaster Road*, 47.

43. Rushdoony, R. J., *The Religion of Revolution*, cited in Wallis, *The Disaster Road*, 68.

44. Eakman, *Cloning of the American Mind*, 232.

45. Cuddy, "Secular humanism in our schools," cited in Wallis, *The Disaster Road*, 58.

46. Eakman, *Cloning of the American Mind*, 255.

47. Cuddy, "Secular humanism in our schools," cited in Wallis, *The Disaster Road*, 55.

48. Dunphy, J., *Humanist*, January-February 1983, 26.

49. Blumenfeld, S. L., *N.E.A.: Trojan Horse in American Education* (Boise, Idaho: The Paradigm Company, 1984).

11.

Man Is More Than an Animal

"What is man, that thou art mindful of him?"

This ancient question, asked by the psalmist 2,500 years ago, has had no lack of attempts to answer. Besides the two views discussed in the previous chapters, that man is an animal—in other words a stimulus-response mechanism—or free and determinant of his own destiny, there are many others. Man is a mere insect, said Francis Church. No, he is great and strong and wise, said Louis Untermeyer. He is a prisoner, said Plato. He is certainly stark mad, maintained Montaigne.[1] He is little lower than the heavenly beings, it is stated in Psalms 8:5.

We could go on, piling up the contrasts and compounding the confusion. But the above should be enough to make the point. The definition of man—or, more exactly, the identity of man—is an open question that has never been settled or agreed upon, and probably never will be. Yet, it is likely that no other question has been more often pondered, debated, wondered at, worried over, and rhapsodized about. The reason is simple: "It is not so much an abstract matter as it sounds at first. The question of man's identity is the most personal of questions. The alternative form of the query 'What is man?' is 'Who am I?' It is not just the 'others out there' but ourselves we are seeking to know when we raise that overwhelming question."[2]

One of the reasons why philosophers fail to find a clear answer to this question can possibly be that they have always attempted to explain man *in terms of* something else. Maybe we must heed the wise counsel of Alexander Pope that "The proper study of mankind is man." Instead of attempting to explain man in terms of something else, it might be more meaningful to explain him in terms of *himself.*

For the purpose of the present deliberation, a possible point of departure to such an approach could perhaps be that we could reword the well-known question of Immanuel Kant. Instead of asking, "What must I *do* to be regarded as a human being?" one could ask, *"What does man need to be fully human?"*

Physical Needs Are Not Man's Only Needs

> Jima Assad sat barefoot in the stifling noontime heat as the sun beat down on her. Her fine black face was drawn and expressionless. There was no more room for emotion, no more strength. This was Sudan, and starvation was on the land. Total, abject, barren misery. Beside Jima lay her son, Nur Allah. The boy was just under two, but his sagging skin, grave eyes and gray complexion made him look like an old man. He was too weak to hold his head up, too weak even to cry.
>
> "Very anemic," nurse Maura Lennon said, leaning over the naked child. "Typical case of advanced malnutrition."[3]

The cause of Nur Allah's problem is that one of his *physical* needs has not been looked after adequately. A lack of food has led to malnutrition. His problem can only be solved by giving him food. For some time, he will also need to receive more food than a normal person does. That will be the only way in which he will be able to regain his normal body weight.

Man's physical needs are of the utmost importance, because physical life must be sustained first. The most important physical needs are: *food, water, oxygen, rest, and protection.* There is also a specific method through which each of these needs is taken care of:

- We must *eat* to satisfy our need for food;
- We must *drink* to satisfy our need for water;
- We must *breathe* to satisfy our need for oxygen;
- We must *sleep* to satisfy our need for rest;
- We must have *shelter* to satisfy our need for protection.

(No hedonistic connotations are to be attached to the above use of the word "satisfy.")

Humans, however, do not only have physical needs. Materialism, and especially the notion of evolution, has blinded social scientists to the fact that man—unlike the animal—has other needs apart from the physical.

The theory of evolution has brought the idea that man can be compared with the animal, even that he *is* an animal. When we compare man and animal from a purely biological perspective, there are no fundamental differences. Man does not possess a single organ, no bone, and no muscle that is not to be found in other vertebrate animals.[4] But because there are similarities, it does not imply, as is often stated, that "*Homo sapiens* is an animal."[5] There are also many dissimilarities. Every morning, millions of people throughout the world get up, dress themselves, eat breakfast and then go to work or to school. In the afternoons they come back home, do homework, eat their supper, sit in front of the TV, go to friends' houses, or read books. Has any person ever seen any animal doing any of these?

One can only wonder when somebody will come up with the brilliant idea that man is actually a plant, on the grounds that there are also similarities between plants and humans. We also have atoms, molecules, and cells in our bodies, just as plants have. We also grow and die, just as plants do, and after death our bodies decay, just as plants do.

The moment man is compared with the animal—and especially when he is reckoned as equal to it—all other aspects and needs regarding man, except the physical, are denied, or they are all reduced to the visible, i.e. the physical. This implies that the possibility that behavior can also be a manifestation of another, invisible aspect of man, is ignored. In the same way that electricity is invisible, but is visibly manifested in a burning light, human behavior can perhaps also be a visible manifestation of other invisible aspects of man. These aspects, which are—since the advent of the notion of evolution—universally ignored, include *the emotional, intellectual, and spiritual*. We have to consider the possibility that the symptoms of ADHD, ODD, and CD—such as that a child does not listen when spoken to, refuses to comply with adults' requests or rules, is hyperactive or impulsive—do not necessarily have a physical cause. These symptoms may simply be a visible manifestation of a child's invisible needs—emotional, intellectual, and spiritual—that have not been adequately attended to.

One can in no way perceive any of these needs in the child—emotional, intellectual, and spiritual—through any of the senses. Evolutionists and materialists will therefore argue that they do not exist. The fact that one cannot see, hear, or feel them, however, does not mean that they do not exist. One cannot see, hear, or feel radio waves. Only the fact that the radio starts playing when you switch it on indicates their existence. One cannot see, hear, or feel X-rays, but one cannot deny their existence when you look at an X-ray photograph.[6] The existence of needs cannot be directly demonstrated, but their existence can be convincingly demonstrated by studying the effect or effects on a person if they were to be neglected or ignored. In the discussions of each of these three invisible needs which follow, we shall therefore not only discuss each need individually, but *also* the effect or effects on a person, especially on a child, if they were to be neglected or ignored.

A person becomes aware of a need only when a deficit is experienced. If you have just had breakfast, you will not be aware of any need for food. Wait a few hours until lunchtime, and your empty stomach will quickly remind you of this need. In the case of Nur Allah, the shortage of food was so severe that it caused him to become visibly undernourished. One can easily imagine his swollen abdomen and emaciated body. Note, however, that he was not inherently ill in any way—he just did not receive enough food.

In the same way, a child, whose emotional needs are not attended to, may become "emotionally undernourished." The child, whose intellectual needs are neglected or ignored, may become "intellectually undernourished," and in the same way a child can also become "spiritually undernourished."

Freedom Without Limits Is No Freedom at All

All human beings have a need for *security, acceptance,* and *dignity.* Just like with the physical needs, there is also a particular method through which each of these emotional needs is satisfied:

- Security is provided through *discipline;*
- *Love* satisfies the need for acceptance;
- Through *respect* it is possible to satisfy the need for dignity.

The method through which security is provided is through discipline. This, unfortunately, is a topic on which there is widespread ignorance in our times, simply because the public, and especially parents, have been deceived about this by psychology and psychiatry in the recent past.

The word discipline means that boundaries are set. These boundaries are set by means of values and norms, and, on a more practical level, by means of rules and regulations. These boundaries set limits to a person's conduct in life ("thou shalt not" do this), but also implies certain obligations ("thou shalt" do that). In the case of a child, the most important persons responsible for enforcing these boundaries are the child's *parents,* or *a parent* in the case of a single parent. Because he has no knowledge of the boundaries, a child cannot set them for himself. As already explained in chapter four, there is nothing that any human being knows, or can do, that he has not learned. Therefore, when a child enters this world, he does not know *that* there are boundaries. He does not know *what* these boundaries are. He does not know *how* to live within these boundaries, and he also has no knowledge of the *consequences,* should he overstep these boundaries. All this he can only learn through *education.*

Being nervous about appearing "too stern" or "authoritarian"— swear words in our modern world—many of today's parents hesitate to set limits or say "no." As Kirkwood remarks, the problem of today's adults is that they wrongly fear that children will dislike them if they impose discipline, and conversely hope children will love them if they act like friends instead of parents and teachers. He states:

> The first thing a child must learn is that being friendly isn't the same as being a friend, and a parent and teacher can't be a friend because the nature of friendship precludes one friend from having authority over another. That's why a buck private in the Army can't be a friend to a four-star general. Friendship blurs the line of authority. And for the same reason generals tell privates what to do, parents must tell children what to do. They know more. Children are not old enough, and don't know enough, to know what they want or need, which is why children are called children and parents are called parents.[7]

Because parents are parents they *must* maintain standards of behavior, and to do this they must be willing to exercise their authority. As Walsh says, the authoritativeness of parents provides the security and sense of direction that children need. And parents *can* set these limits and still keep the lines of communication open.[8]

Little by little, the knowledge of what these boundaries are, how one should live within them and of the consequences one would have to face if one were to deny them, leads to a gradually growing feeling of security in the child. The word "security" comes from the Latin word "securus," meaning "carefree," "without care," "safe," and "secure."

A good example of these meanings of the word can be found in the traffic situation. Because clear boundaries are enforced on drivers by means of strict rules, the motorist has a feeling of security when he drives in his car. As long as everybody accepts these limitations, the motorist can drive his car without worry and with safety and security. However, if there were no traffic rules, or if everybody ignored these rules, there would be total chaos. Nobody would have the freedom to use the roads.

Another example is the sports field, a place where absolute discipline is enforced. The referee will not punish a player for every second or third infringement of a rule; he will punish him immediately. If this were not the case, either the referee's life would be in danger—spectators would probably stone him for being unfair—or the players' lives would be in danger. As players would know that they could take chances, foul play would become commonplace. Games such as American football, rugby, and ice hockey would have been so dangerous that nobody would have had the courage to participate in any of these sports. The strict discipline on the sports field, therefore, gives players the freedom to play free of care, safely and in security.

The word "freedom," however, has acquired a completely unacceptable connotation in recent years. Many people have come to believe that freedom means complete license and total absence of limits. The idea exists that strict rules and regulations are equal to oppressiveness. That the opposite is true can be seen in the traffic situation and on the sports field. Freedom only reigns when there are strict limits that are uniformly enforced.

Nobody can be free if he is not also responsible. To be *responsible* means that a person must be willing to respond to the demand to obey the limits that are set to his behavior. There are billions of people sharing the same world, millions sharing the same country, and often a few sharing the same house. We can only live together in peace and harmony if everybody is willing to accept the responsibility of obeying the boundaries, which brings about certain limitations and obligations. Freedom without limits is *no freedom at all*.

When responsibilities are thrown overboard for the sake of "freedom" and the accompanying notion of "human rights," it can only lead to lawlessness and chaos. In the United States, which is viewed as one of the most liberated nations, at least 1.3 million Americans find themselves behind bars. This means that approximately 519 per one hundred thousand are incarcerated,[9] of which nearly half are violent criminals. In Texas, in 1995, there were 127,000 people in prison. That is nearly equal to the prison population of the whole United States less than 25 years ago.[10]

But this is hardly the full picture. According to a U.S. News and World Report in 1989, 8.1 million serious crimes like homicide, assault, and burglary were committed in a typical year. Only 724,000 adults were arrested and fewer still (193,000) were convicted. Less than 150,000 were sentenced to prison, with thirty-six thousand serving less than a year.[11] A 1987 National Institute of Justice study found that the average felon released due to prison overcrowding commits upwards of 187 crimes per year, costing society approximately $430,000.[12]

Japan, on the other hand, has traditionally been known as a country with a very low crime rate. The streets were described as generally safe, and lost wallets and purses were returned intact to their owners. Tokyo, known as the world's safest major city, suffered muggings in the 1980s at the rate of 40 per year per one million inhabitants. New York City's rate was 11,000.[13] In 1993, the rate of incarceration in Japan was still low—36 per 100,000[14]—compared to America's—more than 500 per 100,000.

But matters in Japan are changing as a juvenile crime wave is spreading across the islands. In the last few years, reports of teen violence, crime, and rising drug use have dominated the media, and a series of school killings have shocked the nation. The first sign that this generation was in serious trouble came in May 1997, when an 11-year-old Kobe boy was decapitated and his head left on a post at his schoolyard gate. The following month, a 14-year-old boy was arrested on suspicion of the crime. It appeared that the boy had killed at least two other schoolchildren. Police attention was drawn to him after he boasted of killing cats, whose severed tongues he carried around in a jar in his pocket.[15]

Reported cases of beatings and other forms of violence committed by schoolchildren at Japanese schools jumped to 29,000 in 1997, up from about 11,000 in 1996.[16] Juveniles committed 44.5 percent of all violent crimes in Japan in 1997.[17] Gang members have an average age of just sixteen and like to mask their faces Lone Ranger-style before setting off to cruise threateningly the nighttime streets of urban Japan, revving up at every opportunity to remind everyone they're there. Their name, with charming Japanese literalness, means "violent running group." Anyone viewed as in their way is liable to get a blow from a baseball bat to the head.[18] Teenage girls from middle-class families prostitute themselves to middle-aged men. Schools, once famous for rigidity and discipline have turned into chaotic places where students even physically assault teachers.[19] Considering the tendency noted in other countries, one could conclude that there is little hope of turning the delinquency tide.

There have been several attempts in the past to explain the tremendous difference in crime rate between the United States and Japan. Of course, such attempts are of great importance. If we could find the *cause* or *causes* for the difference in crime rate between these two countries, we may be able to lay down one or two principles that may be of value. Ignoring the recent surge of youth violence, let us try to find some explanation for the peace that has reigned on the streets of Japan for so long.

One of the reasons that had been suggested in an effort to explain the low crime rate in Japan is the Japanese law forbidding ownership of guns and swords. Besides the police and the military, the only group that is allowed to possess guns are hunters, and such possession is strictly circumscribed.

We have no doubt that gun control in America, or any other country for that matter, will prevent a number of unfortunate incidences. But gun control alone is certainly not the answer. As Dr. Paul Blackman of the National Rifle Association's Institute for Legislative Action points out, gun control in Japan cannot be the *major* cause of their low crime rate. If so, it would be impossible to explain why Japan's non-gun crime rate was so much lower than America's non-gun crime rate. America's non-gun robbery rate in the late 1980s was sixty times that of Japan.[20] One should also not lose sight of the fact that people who are capable of committing crimes with guns are also capable of obtaining illegal guns. Britain is a good example. Despite tight licensing procedures, handgun-related robbery rates in Britain rose about 200 percent during the dozen years before 1996—five times as fast as in the U.S.[21]

Kopel attributed Japan's low crime rates to their superior police work. "Broad powers, professionalism, and community support," as he described it, combined to help Tokyo police solve 96.5 percent of murders, and 82.5 percent of robberies. Compared to these 1980 figures, American police cleared 74 percent of murders, but only a quarter of all robberies. Whereas 70 percent of all Japanese crimes ended in a conviction, only 19.8 percent of American crimes even ended in an arrest. A mere 9 percent of reported American violent crimes ended in incarceration. Compared to the Japanese criminal, the American criminal faced only a minuscule risk of jail. "Is it any wonder that American criminals commit so many more crimes?" Kopel asked.[22]

Civil-rights attorney Kensuke Onuki disagreed with Kopel's description of the Japanese police. He states that the relatively low rate of private criminality in Japan was achieved by "massive police criminality," and compared their law procedures with those used in the film "Midnight Express."[23] As we have little knowledge of the Japanese police's operation procedures, we shall not pronounce judgment upon them. But that a country's police force and law system have much to do with its crime rate, is certain. New York is proof of this. Since toughening its police force and introducing its "zero tolerance" campaign, New York has produced an amazing 50 percent reduction in crime in the last four years. Similarly, when a zero tolerance of crime was launched in 1998 in Huddersfield, as part of Britain's new crime reduction strategy, burglary was cut by 30 percent.[24]

While New York and Huddersfield are seemingly winning their battles against crime, South Africa has gained the unenviable reputation of being one of the most violent and crime-ridden countries in the world. For every one hundred thousand people, more than fifty are murdered per year,[25] a murder rate seven times higher than the United States.[26] Even police are not immune from South Africa's crime wave. The *Mail & Guardian* newspaper in Johannesburg reported that from 1994 to 1998, 240 police officers, on average, were murdered every year. In the United States, which has a population more than six times that of South Africa, the average was 70 police officers murdered each year. In England and Wales, with a combined population 20 percent higher than that of South Africa, the average is fewer than two officers killed per year.[27]

South Africa is the leader in rapes reported—120 per 100,000 residents per year.[28] In the first eleven months of 1998, 14,225 children were reported raped, up from 7,559 reported cases in 1994. Many, however, believe that these official statistics are just the tip of the iceberg. One source estimates that no more than 2.8 percent of all rape cases in South Africa are reported, which would put the total number of women and girls raped each year at more than one million, out of a female population of some 23 million.[29] In a survey, conducted early in 1999 in the South African city of Johannesburg, one in three of the four thousand women questioned by CIET Africa, a nongovernmental organization, said they had been raped in the past year. In a related survey conducted among 1,500 school-children in the Soweto township, a quarter of all the boys interviewed said that "jackrolling"—a South African term for recreational gang rape—was fun. More than half the interviewees insisted that when a girl says "no" to sex, she really means "yes."[30] The public is reminded of this epidemic only when new records are broken, such as the case of a 19-year-old student who was recently attacked and consecutively raped by 15 youngsters. In another case, a 114-year-old woman died after she was pinned to the floor of her township home and assaulted and raped by a 29-year-old man. Even more shocking, perhaps, is the case of four boys, aged seven to nine, who raped a little girl of only two years.

It seems that one is lucky *not* to be a victim in South Africa at some time or other. After the death of Erich Ellmer, for example, the South African-German Chamber of Commerce revealed that of the 30 chief executives of German companies operating in South Africa, 16 had been victims of violent crime.[31] The result has been that many South African homes have been turned into fortresses, with windows and doors girded with iron and with warning signs plastered on surrounding walls. Security companies make a fortune rendering armed response to housebreakings, or selling the latest off-the-wall security systems. Many law-abiding citizens feel that *they* have been incarcerated, while criminals are free.

Considering South Africa's low rates of arrest, conviction, imprisonment, and rehabilitation, it is unlikely that the situation will change in the near future. According to one source, for every thousand crimes committed, 450 are reported, 230 solved, 100 perpetrators prosecuted, 77 convicted, 36 imprisoned and only 8 imprisoned for 2 years or more. Of the 8 imprisoned, 1 will be rehabilitated.[32]

Police can do little to alleviate the crime problem. They are undermanned, undertrained, and underpaid. And according to police sergeant Kriban Naidoo, those are not the only problems. "Our justice system stinks," she said. "What's the use in arresting a man for a crime when he has enough money to hire a fancy lawyer, walk out of court and laugh in your face the next day? What do you do— arrest him, or take his bribe and let him go?"[33]

Considering the comparison between New York and South Africa, it is difficult to deny the role of a country's police force and their law system in upholding social order. Notwithstanding, the Japanese police force is still not the primary reason for Japan's long-existing low crime rate. If so, it would be difficult to explain why

Japanese Americans, who are subjected to American gun regulations and law enforcement, *had an even lower violent crime rate in the 1980s than the Japanese in Japan.*[34] In the same breath one can also ask why *some* of today's children use drugs while others don't, or why *some* are promiscuous while others are not, or why *some* commit crimes while others don't. Drugs are readily available to all, and so are opportunities to be promiscuous or commit crimes.

The reason for Japan's long-standing low crime rate must be sought elsewhere, in all probability in the Japanese culture, more specifically in the *Japanese traditions on child rearing.* If this is a valid explanation for Japan's long-standing low crime rate—and indeed it seems to be the only logical explanation—it suggests that the role of parents is far more powerful than any punitive system can ever be. If parents take their educational task to heart while their children are still young, they can prevent their children from clashing with justice later in their lives.

Unfortunately, Japanese educators have abandoned their traditions on child rearing and now they are paying the price. According to Professor Gentaro Kawakami, Japanese children "don't have a sense of what is wrong and right any more."[35] "Our kids are spoiled," observed another. "Homes [are] a place where children can do anything they want."[36] In addition, focused on economic wealth, Japanese parents have worked for long hours and showered their children with toys and gadgets. But they tend to spend less and less time with their children, alienating them and causing them to feel lonely, which in turn has led many of them to rebel. "This generation doesn't know how to relate to people," says Mariko Kuno Fujiwara, a specialist in youth culture.[37]

Nobody Can Replace a Parent

Social harmony is not established by the presence of armed agents of the law, says Philip Atkinson, but first of all by our *individual attitude toward right and wrong,* which is enforced by our conscience.[38] This attitude toward right and wrong is not an innate quality of a human being, but can only be established by means of proper education. No human being is born with a conscience. A conscience is the result of an established system of decent values and norms, also brought about by proper education.

A child who has been raised without a decent system of values and norms will not develop a conscience. His feelings, urges, and impulses, which may differ from day to day and in accordance with circumstances, are his *only* guidelines to determine his behavior. The problem is that feelings, urges, and impulses do not consider or respect other people, but are always directed only at the person himself. A child who, for example, has an urge to walk around in the classroom, considers neither the teacher who is trying to teach, nor twenty other students, who are trying to learn. He only considers himself.

In contrast to the modern Western lack of consideration and respect for others, an attitude of obedience and impulse control and respect for law and order have always formed an ingrained part of Japanese citizenry for many generations. These values and norms were not genetically transmitted, but had been *taught* to children by their *parents* from mother's breast—also by the Japanese descendants in the United States. In the Japanese culture the role of the parent had always been regarded as very important. Shinichi Suzuki, who earned fame for training thousands of violinists by starting to stimulate them even prior to birth, stated, "The destiny of children lies in the hands of their parents."[39]

Discipline has always played a major role in the Japanese culture. Proper manners were taught at a young age, and parents strictly enforced them. A few that were considered to be important were that children be neat in their appearance, have good posture, be well spoken, and be respectful of their elders. Children were taught to take orders from their elders whether it was an older sibling, adult, parent, or grandparent, but most importantly a male figure. In addition, children, especially girls, were taught to be modest in their behavior, as it was frowned upon when anyone, especially children, acted out or engaged in conflict with others. There were specific roles that were laid out for the children, depending on their gender, age, and birth order. Because all parents taught their children to accept these values, the result was that they, as a society, could live together in harmony.

Japanese society has attached great importance to achievement. Parents put great pressure on their children to excel, not only at school, but also in extracurricular activities such as mastering a musical instrument or performing domestic chores. Teachers in Japanese schools continued with the education of the children along the same lines. Students were reminded of their obligation to family, school, and society. No one suggested that they had rights.[40]

A common perception of Japanese children had always been that they were overly stressed by the strict discipline and the immense academic pressure placed upon them. As already mentioned, they had to cope with a school curriculum that was by far more challenging than the American curriculum.

The image of a stressed out Japanese child may be nothing more than an illusion. Stevenson, Chen and Lee measured the stress levels of eleventh graders in Japan and America. They asked the students, if within the last month:

- They had experienced feelings of stress?
- They had felt depressed?
- They had felt angry?
- They had had difficulty sleeping?
- They had felt nervous while taking a test or getting a test back?

Japanese students reported the lowest occurrence of these characteristics. American students were far likelier to mention feelings of anxiety, stress, or aggression in connection with school. Academic stress was mentioned by 70 percent of American students. The authors noted in their paper that the perception of stressed out Japanese children may be based on informal reports. Until their study, they were unaware of any formal comparative studies. The authors state, "These data do not support the Western stereotype of Asian students as tense young persons driven by relentless pressures for academic excellence. . . . Rather, it was the American students who were more likely to express indications of distress. We believe this occurred because American students do not have a clear idea about the importance they should place on education."[41]

This research confirms once again that discipline leads to security, and not to stress, anger or depression, or to "mental illnesses," as the Mental Hygiene Movement has persuaded millions of parents and teachers to believe. It is the lack of discipline that leads to feelings of insecurity, as well as to many of the so-called mental illnesses—such as ADHD, ODD, and CD.

When consistent discipline is applied, not only does it lead to feelings of security, but it also helps the child to learn self-discipline and self-control. The child learns to set limits to his own behavior and to meet his obligations. However, a child who is allowed to:

- choose for himself what he wants to or does not want to do,
- defy or refuse to comply with adults' requests or rules,
- be a disturbance in the classroom,

- intrude on others or not await his turn,
- be destructive, cruel, aggressive and rebellious, and
- lie, steal, or swear

will not suddenly change once he reaches adulthood. A child who has not been disciplined will become an adult without self-discipline and self-restraint. The saying "as the twig is bent, the tree is inclined" might sound old-fashioned, but it is still valid.

The persons who are responsible for leading the child with discipline to self-discipline and self-restraint are the child's educators, of which the most important are the child's parents. As explained in chapter four, we have no choice about educating and being educated, although we may educate badly and be badly educated. A child can only be well educated if there is firm and loving discipline, so that he can be lead to self-discipline and self-restraint. There is no alternative. Ritalin, Dexedrine, Tegretol, or Catapress cannot do it. A pill cannot satisfy a child's, or an adult's, emotional needs. For that, we need each other. As John Donne expressed it so succinctly more than three centuries ago: "No man is an island." In the case of a child, nobody is more important to look after his emotional needs than his parents.

Unfortunately, few of today's parents realize the importance of their role in the education of their children. When one studies the literature, one soon realizes why this is the case. While on one hand the children are being brainwashed in the classroom to reject their parents' values and norms, on the other hand parents are being brainwashed to believe that they cannot influence their children to accept their values and norms. Harold Koplewicz, author of *It's Nobody's Fault*, reassured parents that some kids have a genetic predisposition or are "hard-wired" for psychiatric disorders and behavioral problems. Judith Rich Harris, author of *The Nurture Assumption: Why Children Turn Out the Way They Do*, went even further. According to Harris it doesn't matter how "good" or "bad" a parent is because a child's development is most influenced by his or her peer groups. She claims there is no proof that parents enjoy more than a genetic influence on how their children turn out and attacks the "nurture assumption," which holds that parents can determine the entire course of their children's lives. This book overflows with such obvious folly that it could easily be dismissed, had it not been published in the prestigious journal *Psychological Review*, endorsed by some of the most respected names in academia and honored by the American Psychological Association.[42]

If one studies the reasons children give as to why they use drugs, one tends to agree with Harris that children are most influenced by their peer groups. The reasons are to "fit in with their friends," to be "accepted by others," to "act cool," and to "see what drugs are like."

If one, however, studies the reasons children give as to why they have decided *not* to use drugs, Harris's theory goes for a loop. In an eight year study of drug/alcohol-free American high school students, the researchers grouped the reasons given by non-using youths into ten "themes." Interestingly, *all* the themes were related to parents and parent involvement. Some of the themes included:

- Non-using students state they have been taught a clear idea of right and wrong—consistently, and from an early age. They also state this concept of right and wrong is modeled by their parents. (The most frequently occurring theme.)
- A large majority of non-using students report that their parents were available to them, particularly during their first eight years. (The second most frequently occurring theme.)
- Nonusers' parents had taught their children that school would be enjoyable and encouraged their children to do well in school. A frequent message is, "you can be anything you want to be, and school is the reason why." (The third most frequently occurring theme.)
- Nonusers describe families that expressed love and affection openly. Hugs, sitting together, and saying "I love you" were common even into the teen years. (The fourth most frequently occurring theme.)
- Nonusers describe parents who agreed on discipline and who were consistent in its implementation. The majority describes their parents as strict, fair, and predictable. (The sixth most frequently occurring theme.)
- Nonusers enjoy being at home. They talk of an atmosphere where "kids are wanted." Rules exist, but rules also allow friends to be welcome and permission for safe fun. (The seventh most frequently occurring theme.)[43]

If this doesn't strike you, it certainly struck us. What struck us especially was that love earned fourth place, while the so-called cause of "mental illnesses," knowing right from wrong, came out on top. What more evidence does one need that parents, *and* discipline, are of the utmost importance. The question to be answered is therefore not whether to discipline or not, but rather *how* to discipline, in other words, how does one teach a child to accept the "thou shalt nots" and the "thou shalts."

The Three Cornerstones of Discipline

The first cornerstone of proper discipline is that parents should lead by *example*. We as parents would have little credibility if we tried to teach our children to act in one way, while we acted in another. If we cursed and swore everyday, we could not expect of them *not* to do the same. In fact, in all probability, cursing and swearing is what they will do. Deeds count more than words.

This, however, does not imply that words are worthless. By means of *instruction*, which implies intentional or purposeful teaching, a child is taught what his limitations and obligations are, and of the consequences, should he ignore these boundaries. By being told what he should do and what not, a child learns that he should respect authority as well as other people and that friendliness, thankfulness, honesty, truthfulness, and unselfishness are priceless virtues. Through instruction, a child also learns that lying and stealing are wrong and that sexual dissoluteness and drug abuse lead to self-destruction. The teaching of all these values and norms are a parent's responsibility, and cannot be left to the school, or to any other person or institution. In fact, in this respect the Bible gives parents a direct command. Read Deuteronomy 6:4-7 and you will find:

> These commandments that I give you today are to be upon your hearts. Impress them on your children. Talk about them when you sit at home and when you walk along the road, when you lie down and when you get up. Tie them as symbols on your hands and bind them on your foreheads. Write them on the door frames of your houses and on your gates.

Similar instructions are given to parents in Proverbs 22:6, "Train the child in the way he should go," and in Ephesians 6:4, "bring them up in the training and instruction of the Lord."

To discipline a child by means of instruction unfortunately requires *time*, a commodity that very few children are granted by their parents today. Not many parents are willing to step out of the rat race and spend time with their children. According to one study, the average American child watches four hours of TV per day—a total of 1,680 minutes per week—while parents spend only thirty-nine minutes per week in meaningful conversation with their children.[44]

Should we find it a source of wonder then that so many of today's children have gone astray? As Walsh correctly states:

> We adults need to examine our priorities in terms of how we spend our time. . . . [K]ids need more time with adults who care about them. The term "quality time" has worked its way into our contemporary vocabulary to rationalize the lack of "quantity time," but our kids need both. . . . Kids need guidance, nurturing, reassurance, and direction from parents, and they can get it only through a lot of interaction and communication. Kids can't grow up on automatic pilot—they need and deserve the active participation of adults in their lives.[45]

A good example and proper instruction, however, is not the end of the story. Being a parent is unfortunately not *that* simple. In exchange for the tremendous joy that parenthood can provide, we have to work much harder than this. The challenging part of parenthood is that *no* child will accept all the limitations and obligations imposed on him. At some time or other, any child *will* defy the authority of his parents by deliberately overstepping the boundaries that have been set for him. Thereby he tests these boundaries, as well as the authority of his parents. *All* children do this, some more often than others. Children have always done this, and they always will. In fact, there is *no* human being that is not guilty of deliberately overstepping the boundaries from time to time. We all know what the speed limits are. We all know what a stop sign means. Yet there are many drivers who break these rules at some time or other. There are, of course, also those who, although they may not be guilty of breaking traffic rules, may be "creative" when completing their tax returns.

The reason for this is simple. We are *human*. However great man's need for security, folly is and will always be part of human nature. This quality of man we could already observe in Adam and Eve. God had told them they could eat *anything* in the Garden *except* the forbidden fruit ("do not pass this boundary"). Yet they challenged the authority of the Almighty by deliberately disobeying His command. Solomon, in his wisdom, said, "There is not a righteous man on earth who does what is right and never sins" (Eccles. 7:20). The well-known dictum of Paul also serves as a confirmation of man's sinful nature: "For what I do is not the good I want to do; no, the evil I do not want to do—this I keep on doing" (Rom. 7:19). A parent's responsibility is thus not to liberate his child from his sinful nature—simply because it cannot be done. However, it is certainly his responsibility to drive *enough* folly out of his child's heart so that he will eventually be able to lead a virtuous and decent life, and not be a murderer, rapist, robber, drug addict, or alcoholic. As Ashley Montagu said, the wonder of the baby lies in its promise, a promise that can only come true with the required help and assistance. Viewed differently, there are two possibilities locked in every child: there is the ugly, bad, and evil possibility, but there is also the beautiful, noble, and good possibility. Due to the sinful nature of man, the evil possibility will come true by itself, but the good possibility must be *made to come true*. This can only be accomplished by means of education, and an important ingredient of this education is discipline.

The necessity of discipline cannot be emphasized enough. Its presence builds nations, while its absence causes nations to crumble. The mighty Roman Empire, for example, was built up through cast-iron discipline. One of the most important reasons for its downfall was the fact that all values and norms were thrown overboard. The enormous moral decay that occurred during the end of the Roman Empire's existence is clearly reflected in their literature, in their amusements, and in their life-styles, all of which included extravagant sex and violence.

Discipline is important for the survival of a society or a nation. Secondly, the rules, regulations, and laws imposed by a country's government provide security for its citizens. If there were no laws, or if these laws were too slack or were not enforced strictly, a country's citizens would experience a lack of security. In the same way, parental discipline determines, to a great extent, the emotional security of an individual child. Without discipline, or without proper discipline, he will have no emotional security.

There is, however, yet another purpose for parental discipline—one that is futuristic in nature. This future purpose is to enable the child to eventually lead a virtuous and decent life as an adult. As Goethe stated so wisely many years ago, "If we take man as he is, we make him worse; if we take him as he ought to be, we help him become it."[46] Perhaps Goethe derived this wisdom from Proverbs 22:6. In this verse, parents are instructed to "Train the child in the way he should go," because, if they do, the outcome will be that ". . . when he is old he will not turn from it."

Due to the moral decay all around us, many parents seem to regard this purpose of discipline as an impossible mission. We disagree. We agree that it may be a lot more difficult than it used to be before psychology and psychiatry came on the scene, but we shall never accept that this futuristic purpose is impossible. Although we disagree with some of the traditional Japanese disciplinary measures, the Japanese Americans nevertheless provide proof that, even in the midst of a crumbling society, children *can* still be reared to be virtuous and decent. The above-mentioned study of drug/alcohol-free American high school students also provides proof of this.

When parents are asked what their prospects for their children are, one usually receives answers such as, "that they will be happy," "that they will be successful," or "that they will achieve academically." The problem is that none of these prospects are likely to come true if the child does not know how to lead a virtuous and decent life. A drug addict will not be happy, successful, or achieve academically. A person who leads a virtuous and decent life, on the other hand, has the prospects of happiness, success, and academic achievement. If we, as parents, make the *right* choices for our children, many other bonuses can and will probably be added to their lives. Solomon made the right choice. He chose wisdom rather than a long life, wealth, or the death of his enemies. God not only gave him the requested wisdom, but also riches and honor, as well as the prospect of a long life if he were to continue obeying God's statures and commands (1 Kings 3:7-14). In the well-known fairy tale of King Midas, on the other hand, the king made the wrong choice by choosing wealth. Very soon he had to give up his wealth to save his daughter when she, and all his worldly possessions, had also turned into gold.

When a parent is thus confronted by a child who, despite a good example and proper instruction, deliberately oversteps the boundaries that have been set to him, the parent has no choice but to take action. As we have seen from the statistics cited in the first chapter, imaginative labels such as ADHD, ODD, or CD will not solve the problem. These labels, at best, sidestep the problem in the short term, but are likely to have destructive results in the long term.

Taking action when a child deliberately oversteps the limits set to him inevitably implies that he must be *punished*. Thereby we arrive at one of the most controversial issues of modern times: *whether* a child should be punished at all, and if so, *what method* should be used to punish him. Thousands of books and articles, with opinions of experts that differ widely and violently from each other, have been published and are still being published annually, thereby contributing to the growing confusion that exists among parents on this matter. Although it is an alarming fact that there are millions of parents who are indifferent, even apathetic toward their children, there are undoubtedly also millions of parents who want only the best for the children in their care. For these parents, a final resolution on this issue is becoming ever more pressing. For parents who are already fighting a losing battle with children who are uncontrollable, finality on the matter is even more important, as their children are particularly in danger of going astray in the future.

Because the evolutionist view of man considers man to be fundamentally good, the idea that a child should be punished is rejected. According to this view, man is innocent and not, as the Bible states, conceived and born in sin. In the education of the child, according to the evolutionist approach, it is believed that the parent should not try to change the child in any way, but should just allow whatever is in the child to develop freely. Parents should not impose boundaries upon their children, because their children should be free to express themselves and learn through their own experiences. A parent does not have to punish his child, because it is believed that the natural consequences of the child's actions will discipline him so that he will be able to apply self-discipline in the future.

It is unfounded notions like these that can be held responsible for the present chaos in education and for the destruction of our children. If we consider as an example just the last of the above misconceptions, it would be difficult to explain why children continue to commit the same misdeeds. The following case serves to illustrate this:

> For as long as Vicky and George Browne [not their real names] can remember, their son, Gary, has been a different and difficult child. At age 3, he was already stubborn, resistant to discipline and hyperactive. After he started school, teachers constantly complained that he cursed, shoved, and punched classmates. In grades 5 and 6, he was expelled several times.
>
> Now 13, Gary is in a special junior-high class for students with learning and behavioral difficulties. He has no friends and, since he was kicked off the hockey team last year for brawling, he has hung out with a gang of trouble-prone 16- and 17-year-olds. He sometimes smokes, drinks and uses marijuana. He has tried LSD. Recently, he was caught shop-

lifting.

The advocates of childrearing practices based on evolutionist notions are unable to explain such repeated misdeeds according to their theories, and in an effort to sweep such obvious flaws in their theories under the carpet, they fabricated all kinds of disorders and syndromes. In the case of Gary, it is also the case. The article continues:

> Gary's problem, called antisocial behavior or a *conduct disorder* (our italics), is the most serious, occurring in about 6 percent of youngsters. Typically, they always break the rules, are chronically aggressive and have explosive uncontrollable tempers. They're mean to people and animals. They lie and cheat.[47]

Behaviorism, also founded on an evolutionist view of man, has since the 1930s brought with it the idea that a child who does something wrong or behaves badly should be ignored. If, however, he behaves well, he must receive attention. If a child, for example, throws a temper tantrum, the parent should withdraw himself and go to another room. As soon as the child has calmed down, the parent should reward him for his calm behavior—perhaps with a cookie or something. In this way—it is assumed—the child will learn to behave in an acceptable manner. The behaviorists hit upon this peculiar idea by observing mice running in mazes. A mouse, they discovered, learns much faster if the experimenter rewards his correct turns, than when his incorrect choices are punished with a mild electric shock. From this and similar studies have come the assumption that punishment has little influence on human behavior.[48]

As already stated at the beginning of this chapter, there are radical differences between man and animal. Children are not mice. A child is capable of rebellious and defiant attitudes that have no relevance to a puzzled mouse sitting in a maze. Of course punishment will not teach a child something that he cannot do—and punishment may also never be used for this purpose—but it definitely helps to keep a child within the boundaries of acceptable behavior, on condition that the boundaries are already known to him. Such punishment, in collaboration with the other two cornerstones of discipline, will eventually help the child to acquire self-discipline and self-restraint.

If it were true that unacceptable behavior would decrease when it is ignored, traffic officers should start ignoring drunken drivers and people who exceed the speed limit. Referees should start ignoring foul play on the sports fields. And, remember that, when a burglar breaks into your house, you should ignore him! Remember also that you give him a lot of attention if you should meet him on the street the next day. In that way, according to the behaviorists, you will certainly teach him never to break into your house again, and we should soon live in a crime-free and problem-free society.

Leonardo da Vinci had certainly not heard about mice in mazes when he wrote, "He who does not punish evil commands it to be done."[49]

Notes

1. Matson, F. W., *The Idea of Man* (New York: Dell Publishing Co., Inc., 1976), xiii.

2. Ibid., xiii-xiv.

3. Chelminski, R., "Africa's man-made famine," *Reader's Digest*, vol. 140, 1992.

4. Vloemans, A., *De Mens als Waagstuk* (Den Haag: H. P. Leopolds Uitgevers-mij N. V., 1949).

5. Midgley, M., *Beast and Man: The Roots of Human Nature* (Hassocks, Sussex: The Harvester Press, 1978).

6. De Beer, G. P., Atomic Energy Corporation of S.A., personal conversation.

7. Kirkwood, R. C., "Best friends worst parents," *The Ottawa Sun*, 26 January 1999, 15.

8. Walsh, D., *Selling Out America's Children: How America Puts Profits before Values—And What Parents Can Do* (Minneapolis: Fairview Press, 1995).

9. Mauer, M., "America behind bars: The international use of incarceration." *The Sentencing Project*, September 1994.

10. "Imprisonment is not the answer," www. strenghtech.com.

11. *U.S. News and World Report*, 31 July 1989.

12. "10 Myths of gun control," *NRA Institute for Legislative Action*, March 1996.

13. Kopel, D. B., "Japanese gun laws and crime," *American Rifleman*, December 1988.

14. Mauer, "America behind bars."

15. Parry, R. L., "Rabbit killer makes Japan's parents fear for children," *Independent*, 9 September 1997, 10.

16. "Police say serious crime by young Japanese up sharply," *The Associated Press*, 22 December 1998.

17. Jones, G., "Japanese fear economy not sole problem: Crime, scandal, suicides adding to country's woes," *The Dallas Morning News*, 22 July 1999, 1A.

18. Kramer, G., "Mad in Japan," *Independent on Sunday*, 7 June 1998, 5.

19. Larimer, T., et al., "Young Japan: From we to me with its in-your-face style and endless thirst for thrills, Japan's new generation wants to transform the nation," *Time*, 3 May 1999, 18+.

20. Kopel, "Japanese gun laws and crime."

21. "10 Myths of gun control," *NRA Institute for Legislative Action*.

22. Kopel, "Japanese gun laws and crime."

23. "How does Japan get that low crime rate, anyway?" *Los Angeles Times*, website.

24. *BBC News*, 29 September 1998.

25. Susman, T., "United in anger over crime: S. Africa's suspects get zero tolerance," *Newsday*, 23 May 1999, A19.

26. "African police custody deaths high," *The Atlanta Journal*, 22 May 1998, C02.

27. Melvin, D., "Crime mars ANC's political record," *The Atlanta Constitution*, 27 May 1999, A14.

28. "Violence explodes in the Cape of murder," *Cape Argus*, 2 April 1998.

29. Olojede, D., "Silent no more: Victim sheds light on rampant rape in South Africa," *Newsday*, 31 January 1997, A05.

30. *BBC News*, 19 January 1999.

31. "Where violence comes by day and night," *Newspaper Publishing P.L.C.*, 1996.

32. "Nedcor Project on crime, violence and investment," website.

33. Melvin, "Crime mars ANC's political record."

34. Kopel, "Japanese gun laws and crime."

35. "Crime hits postwar record in Japan," *United Press International,* 13 October 1998.

36. Kirkwood, "Best friends worst parents."

37. Larimer, et al., "Young Japan."

38. Atkinson, P., "A study of our decline," 1998, www.users.bigpond.com/smartboard/decline/civwot/htm.

39. Suzuki, S., *Nurtured by Love: A New Approach to Education* (New York: Exposition Press, 1969).

40. Rohlen, T. P., *Japan's High Schools* (Berkeley: University of California Press, 1983).

41. Stevenson, Chen & Lee, "Mathematics achievement of Chinese, Japanese and American children: Ten years later," 1996, www.redshift.com/~jmichael/html/stress.html.

42. Rubin, B. M., "Do parents make a difference?" *St. Louis Post-Dispatch,* 16 September 1998, E4.

43. "Why kids don't use drugs," *District 66 Community Update,* April 1990.

44. The Brown University child and adolescent behavior letter, website.

45. Walsh, *Selling Out America's Children.*

46. Frankl, V. E., *Psychotherapy and Existentialism* (Harmondsworth, Middlesex: Penguin Books, 1973), 23.

47. Katz, S., "New help for troubled kids," *Chatelaine,* vol. 67, 1 September 1994, 92-96.

48. Dobson, J., *The Strong-Willed Child* (Eastbourne: Kingsway Publications, 1993), 36.

49. Ibid., 37.

12.

Training for
Self-discipline and Self-restraint

If a defiant and disobedient child needs to be punished with the ultimate object of leading him to become an adult with self-discipline and self-restraint, then the first question would naturally be what *method* will be effective in accomplishing this task? If one studies the literature on this topic, one is simply inundated by a deluge of conflicting ideas, arguments and research results. If one analyzes these conflicting ideas, however, one soon discovers that the wrangling is mainly between two parties, the one endorsing corporal punishment/spanking, and the other opposing it.

Until a few decades ago, corporal punishment/spanking was believed to be the most effective punishment for defiant children. "Spare the rod and spoil the child" was a common saying and, as seen in the following report in the *Reader's Digest* of May 1963, the virtues of this time-honored method were unequivocally proclaimed:

> The bailiff rapped for order in the city court of the small industrial community of Whiting, Ind. Judge William Obermiller glanced at the youths, aged 15 to 20, whose names led the docket. They were slouched in a defiant row. Police had arrested them at a beer party on the town's Lake Michigan beach just as they began an unprovoked attack on three passersby. All the boys had records of minor delinquency—loitering, truancy and fighting. Their friends sat in the back of the court, grinning, waiting to see the defendants put this judge in his place.

> On the bench, Judge Obermiller studied their soiled records, then their soiled faces. Brassily, they returned his look. All of the boys, he observed, wore black leather jackets with broad belts, combs sticking out of breast pockets like badges, long, greasy ducktail haircuts.

"These defendants are not prepared for trial," the judge announced at last. "Bailiff, take them to a barber."

Across the street, two barbers started snipping to Judge Obermiller's specifications. "Make them short," he directed. "Make them GI."

Judge Obermiller first received notice outside his own community last year when the juvenile court referred to him four boys, two 16, one 15, one 17, charged with fighting, hit-and-run with a borrowed car, and being drunk in public. After the quartet had swaggered into court, the 15-year-old insolently leaned an elbow on the bench, pulled a roll of bills from his pocket and spoke sharply to the judge. "Okay," he said. "What's the fine? How much do you want?"

"Sit down," Obermiller directed the boy. He turned to the rest of the court. "This case is continued until next Thursday evening," he said. "And, bailiff, I want the parents of these four boys to appear here with them."

Thursday night the surly quartet again stomped up to the bench. When the youngest barked an impudent reply to the judge's first question and his mother remonstrated quietly, the son snapped at her, "Shut up!" Judge Obermiller half rose from his seat, then settled back, looking grim.

"How long since you spanked this boy?" he inquired of the father. "Never? You never spanked him?"

Then, addressing the bailiff, the judge said, "Have the officers turn the boy over and hold him, bottom-up. Then spank him—hard—with your bare hand. Give him 15 whacks. Maybe that will teach him not to sass his mother."

While the policemen held the squirming youth, the bailiff spanked as directed. Judge Obermiller glanced around the courtroom. The young ruffians who had come to see their gang hero put the law in its place were sneaking quietly away.

The four boys answered questions respectfully the rest of that evening. They were put on probation, ordered to report regularly to the judge. According to Whiting school superintendent G. O. Burman, three of these four are "showing great scholastic improvement and are settling down, causing no trouble in their classes." The fourth boy has moved away, and Whiting has no report on his progress.[1]

One can talk to practically anyone from the "old school" and they will tell you similar stories that confirm the effectiveness of the "rod of reproof." In a letter to a South African newspaper, a certain Mr. Van der Merwe writes about a magistrate M. J. Bestbier, with whom he used to work in the 1950s. In those days an accused of eighteen years or under could be sentenced to ten lashes with a light cane. If there was any doubt about the age of the accused, it was recorded as eighteen and the magistrate would sentence him to ten lashes with the cane. It seemed to work well, testifies Van der Merwe, as the crime rate in the district dropped by 50 percent during the two years he worked with Bestbier, from about 5,000 cases per year to less than 2,500.[2]

When recalling the past, one would hear some people say things like "I wish I had a dime for every time I got a whipping. I'd be rich." Others would tell you, "I used to get a whipping at school and get whipped again when I got home."[3] Terms like "brutality and abuse," that one frequently encounters these days when some people refer to corporal punishment, are never used by those reminiscing about the "good old days." In fact, as the following letter of Richard Miller shows, a hymn of praise is usually sung to the individuals who administered the whippings:

> What is wrong with the fathers of this state? First, you read about boys wanting to kill their school principal and fellow classmates. Then, you read in the paper about boys chasing a 73-year-old man out of his home and doing damage to it and also raping some girls ("More arrests sought in Madison crime spree," Nov. 21).
>
> Don't the fathers believe in using discipline on their boys any more? Fathers now should have what my father had when I was small, as did most fathers at the time: a razor strop, which was used for something more than sharpening a razor.
>
> You would try something like these boys did, and it wouldn't take long for my father to get that strop off of the hook and lay it on your bottom good and hard. It sure would make you think twice before doing something again.
>
> I know people will say, "Oh, that is child abuse." My father did not abuse me. He was trying to teach me to be a decent

person and not one to cause trouble. I don't believe in child abuse. I would never want anybody to abuse a child.

But not believing in spanking a child is foolish. A good spanking didn't hurt us when we were small and it sure isn't going to hurt anybody now.

That strop hurt like blazes when it was laid on me, but it taught me to respect my parents, teachers and everybody else. Maybe it is time for fathers to get back to the old days and get a strop in their house and use it when it is needed.[4]

If one reads articles and letters such as the above, it is hard to understand why so much suspicion is being cast on this time-honored tradition. In fact, suspicion seems to be a mild word. There are many people nowadays who violently oppose the idea of spanking a child. "I am really disappointed to read the opinions of all those who are in favor of spanking," one mother responded to a recent Internet poll entitled *To spank or not to spank:*

I shudder when other parents say "I was spanked as a child, and I thank my parents." I don't see much difference between that and battered women who feel they deserve to be beaten. It makes me sick. Lots of people have said there is a difference between being spanked and beaten. What, exactly, is the difference? Is it the velocity of your hand/belt/hairbrush/etc. . . . as it hits your child's backside? Or is it the place on the child's body you're actually hitting? Or is it the number of times you actually hit? In my opinion, spanking is a "nice" word people give to a violent practice. I believe that spanking is a stupid, lazy response to children's misbehaving.

The majority of today's experts on child education would undoubtedly agree with the above-quoted anti-spanking mom—especially Murray A. Straus, who authored the book *Beating the Devil out of Them* in 1994. His work is most frequently quoted in recent times to call this method of punishment in question. According to Straus (1) all the really violent societies in the world allow corporal punishment of children; (2) the greater the degree of approval of corporal punishment in a state, the higher the murder rate; (3) the more corporal punishment in schools, the higher the rate of violence among students; (4) the more corporal punishment in middle childhood or early adolescence, the greater the probability of crime and delinquent behavior; (5) corporal punishment is associated with poor interpersonal and managerial skills, depression, suicide, and alcohol abuse; (6) more corporal punishment means a lower likelihood of graduating from college; (7) corporal punishment increases the risk of becoming a generally angry person; and (8) the more corporal punishment a man experienced the more likely he is to beat his wife.[5]

Other adverse effects, often claimed by anti-spanking activists, is that spanking on the buttocks can create an association between pain and pleasure in the child's mind, and lead to sexual difficulties in adulthood. "Spanking wanted" advertisements in alternative newspapers are frequently cited to make the point.

According to Farrell, an advocate of spanking, much of the writings of the anti-spanking league "reveal little evidence, much opinion, and a good deal of exaggeration and moralizing."[6] And, their arguments are fraught with illogicalities, Farrell might have added.

The Illogicalities of the Humanists

According to the logic of anti-spankers, the first half of the twentieth century should have been a hellish period of violent crime in America, as more than 90 percent of American parents spanked their children then. Notably, it is the *second* half of the twentieth century that is characterized by violent crime, a trend that had its onset at the same time that American psychiatrists and psychologists began to cast doubt upon this time-honored tradition. Influenced by these experts, many parents have abandoned this tradition in favor of modern disciplinary practices, such as the withdrawal of privileges or taking "time-out." Many parents who spank their children today do so only as a last resort—when all else has failed. A survey of American parents shows a drop in the use of spanking as the main disciplinary method from 59 percent in 1962 to 19 percent in 1993. In the same period, corporal punishment in schools has been outlawed in many American states. Even in states where it has not been outlawed, school principals are often reluctant to administer this kind of discipline, fearing that it could land them in legal trouble.

The tendency of violence to *increase* when corporal punishment/spanking is questioned or outlawed is mirrored in other countries. The Swedish government outlawed spanking in 1979 and started an extensive education program to wean parents away from this form of punishment. Since the ban, police reports of teen violence have soared sixfold in the following decade. "What is happening in Sweden is gang violence—mobbing as they call it over there," Dr. Robert Larzelere reported on the Swedish situation a decade after the banning.[7]

In Britain, corporal punishment was outlawed in schools by the 1986 Education Act after a 1982 ruling by the European Court of Human Rights. Ten years later, in 1996, three newspaper polls showed that two-thirds of the people wanted corporal punishment to be reinstated. This change of heart was brought about by the "breakdown of discipline in schools and order on streets,"[8] and the "growing violence among young boys."[9] The Ridings School in Halifax, for example, was closed by the local authorities after reports of assaults on teachers. The *Daily Telegraph* told stories of fights in classrooms, of teachers being bombarded with fireworks and spittle. One 14-year-old boy boasted that he had set fire to a window frame with a cigarette lighter. This is the sort of behavior that has led teachers at the school to ask for the expulsion of sixty "hard-core" troublemakers—about 10 percent of the pupils.[10] Another newspaper reported a woman teacher of this school being sexually assaulted while a male teacher was punched in the face.[11]

In New Zealand, corporal punishment was outlawed in public schools in 1990. Violence, however, did not decrease. In fact, a 1997 report stated that 70 percent of secondary school teachers in New Zealand had been assaulted physically by a student in the previous year.[12]

In South Africa, corporal punishment in schools was abolished in 1996. Less than a year later, the *Cape Argus* published an article warning that action is needed urgently to prevent playing fields turning into "battlegrounds." In one case, a twelfth grade student and martial arts expert hit a younger boy so hard that he had to have reconstructive surgery. At another school, a boy cutting in line at the snack bar during break was stabbed with a bread knife. Violence "became fashion overnight," one principal said. "Bring back corporal punishment. A good whack or two on the behind is not child abuse or violence, it is just effective punishment."[13]

At Manenberg Senior Secondary School in South Africa, where pupils have manhandled teachers, the principal, Abdurahman Petersen, says the abolition of corporal punishment has tied the hands of teachers and brought about mayhem:

> Taking away corporal punishment is a disservice to children, and to education as a whole. We have to call in parents every

time children get unruly. We detain them [the children], but
this does not work on many occasions. The children defy us
because they know there is nothing we can do. Sometimes
we suspend unruly children, but this is a tragedy because it
deprives the child of an education. Discipline fell away after
corporal punishment was abolished last year. The boys swear
at and manhandle women teachers. If a child knows they
can be punished, they will behave much better.[14]

Except for the abolition of corporal punishment in the schools,
the majority of South African parents have abandoned spanking as
a disciplinary practice in favor of American practices, such as the
withdrawal of privileges or taking "time-out." Those who still cling
to this tradition are frequently ridiculed in the press. They are continually reminded that times have changed. They are right, times
have changed, but children—obviously—have not. Without the "rod
of reproof" many act like little vandals, having no respect for other
people or their property.

The situation in Japan is somewhat different. Although corporal punishment in schools is legally prohibited in Japan—the first
law prohibiting it was passed in 1879, repealed in 1885, reinstated
in 1890, repealed again in 1900, and once again reinstated in 1941—
the hickory stick was still much in use in Japanese schools by the
end of the 1970s. While Americans were debating classroom discipline at that time, many believing that sparing the rod was *saving*
the child, there was not much debate in Japan.[15]

An increasing number of disciplinary actions against Japanese
teachers, however, have caused this practice to be gradually phased
out. In 1996, a record number of teachers were disciplined for inflicting corporal punishment on their students. A total of 436 teachers at public schools were subjected to disciplinary measures ranging
from suspensions to pay cuts,[16] which have brought this practice to
a halt. While the age-old concept of *konjo*—as it is called—was
losing its place in the classroom, discipline in Japanese homes was
going astray at the same time. The result is telling. One Japanese
teacher described how one of her students broke windows, hit other
children, spat on the floor, and even urinated publicly. Other kids
fidget, chatter incessantly, leave class without permission and won't
help clean up the classroom. Things are so bad one local government sent a letter to parents reminding them to teach children
manners and obedience. This is once again evidence of a startling
development in a society once known for its courtesy, deference to

legitimate authority, obedience, and manners.[17]

The logic of anti-spankers should also imply that countries such as Singapore and Brunei would swarm with hard criminals. In both countries caning is not used only for children, but also for adult lawbreakers. Modern Singapore provides an extreme example of a spanking society. In the home, most Singaporean parents cane their children and strongly approve of physical discipline. In schools, headmasters physically discipline unruly delinquents, and Singapore still whips adults in its criminal justice system.[18] The laws in Singapore are strict and punishment severe. Its paternalistic government strictly enforces laws that prohibit pornography and ban smoking, eating, chewing gum, or drinking in designated public places. It is even illegal to fail to flush a toilet. The possession of drugs is punishable by death, and being caught for vandalism or rape can lead to a jail sentence, a fine, *and* caning.

According to the logic of anti-spankers, Singapore should be the most violent society on earth, a world where life is "solitary, poor, nasty, brutish, and short." Yet Singapore is one of the most nonviolent of all industrialized societies. In Singapore, women walk the streets freely without fear of being mugged, assaulted, raped, or robbed. Children are well-behaved and respectful, vandalism and juvenile delinquency are rare, and Singaporean schoolchildren perform remarkably well on international measures of academic achievement.[19] Hopefully, Singaporean parents will continue in their ways and not follow in the footsteps of the Japanese.

The laws in Brunei are equally strict and punishment equally severe. Under the current law, for example, possession of heroin and morphine derivatives of more than fifteen grams, or cannabis of more than twenty grams, carries the death sentence. Possession of lesser amounts carries a minimum twenty year jail term *and* caning. The result, as in the case of Singapore, is a low crime rate, and rare occasions of violent crime. (As psychology was introduced at the University of Brunei Darussalam in 1998, it may be interesting to see what happens to Brunei's crime rate over the next few decades.)

The problem with some researchers is that they will "find" what they are looking for. If they *want* to prove that corporal punishment leads to violence, that is what they *will* prove, no matter how they have to twist the facts and no matter how much their "findings" are contradicted by evidence from real life. The reason why they would deliberately fake research on this subject is obvious. If *correctly* applied, corporal punishment/spanking is an effective tool in maintaining order at home and in the classroom (discipline in the here and now), and also in teaching children right from wrong (which eventually leads to self-discipline). As Proverbs 22:15 states, "Folly is bound up in the heart of a child, but the rod of discipline will drive it far from him." As it is the goal of the humanists either to create chaos, or to free man from concepts of right and wrong, they have everything to gain by proving that corporal punishment is destructive.

The story of Cyril Burt, England's first true psychologist, and one of its most distinguished ones, should serve as a warning to parents against too readily accepting the scientific findings of psychology and psychiatry. Burt's research on inherited intelligence proved that intellect is born, not made. His scientific findings were mainly based on large-scale studies comparing the intelligence quotient (IQ) scores of identical twins and nonidentical twins, and identical twins that had been reared apart. His work became the cornerstone of all theories of inherited intelligence, helped shape the British school system, and was considered of such consequence that, in 1946, Burt became the first psychologist to be knighted. And yet, within a year of his death, his methods, data, and honesty were in serious question. A horrified psychological community discovered that much of Burt's work rested on data that had been doctored and possibly made up. In fact, it appeared that Burt used perhaps up to twenty pseudonyms (names that he had invented) to promote his own journal.[20]

Burt's case is also not an isolated case. In 1988, as a further example of the readiness of psychologists to twist the facts, psychologist Stephen Breuning, an expert in the study of hyperactivity and mentally retarded children, pleaded guilty of falsifying data that he presented to the federal agency funding his research. This case is particularly serious because Breuning's research had a rapid impact on the choice of drugs used to treat certain behavioral disorders in mentally retarded children. As Robert Sprague, his accuser, put it, "the issue of scientific fraud in research on psychotropic medications . . . is not an academic game, but directly influences the lives and welfare of tens of thousands of mentally retarded people."

After reading Martin Gardiner's *Fads and Fallacies in the Name of Science* (published by Dover Publications, 1957), and also through our own research, it gradually became evident to us that people can be persuaded remarkably easily to accept and follow even the most illogical and clearly unproven ideas. *Gullibility,* it seems, is the biggest qualitative difference between man and animal. Nothing could ever persuade a lion that he is *not* a lion. Nothing could ever persuade a monkey *not* to be a monkey. Nothing could ever persuade an ant that he is anything *but* an ant. It took only *one* book, however, that of Darwin, to persuade millions of people that they are animals. Likewise, millions of parents were willing to abandon tried and tested traditions and the experience of parents over thousands of years in favor of totally unproven new and modern psychological ideas on child rearing. Have these modern views managed to make the world any better? The answer is a very emphatic NO. As more and more parents follow psychological gimmicks such as ignoring misbehavior and rewarding good behavior, withdrawing privileges and "time-out," youth-related problems are becoming more and more acute. At the same time, homes are being transformed into stressful places. Many of today's parents are worn-out by their children's continuous misbehavior, some are forced to isolate themselves to avoid embarrassment in public, while others are afraid—and even terrified—of their own children.

Perhaps we should take the story of Elijah and the prophets of Baal to heart. The prophets of Baal could not set the wood beneath the sacrifice on fire, even though they shouted, danced, prophesied frantically and slashed themselves with swords and spears until the blood flowed. When Elijah prayed to the true God, however, the "fire of the Lord fell and burned up the sacrifice, the wood, the stones and the soil, and also licked up the water in the trench" (1 Kings 18:38). So far, nothing positive has come from the alien methods of psychology and psychiatry. The only visible result of all the frantic shouting, dancing, and prophesying of psychologists and psychiatrists, and of all their pills and potions, is just that it is utterly destroying all children. So, perhaps we should follow the ways of the Lord again, and we might discover a light burning in our children's hearts. Our old-fashioned forefathers relied on Him. They used His Word as the instruction manual in the education of their children. Although our forefathers were certainly not perfect, the truth remains that they were many times more successful in turning their children into adults with self-discipline and self-restraint. Such an outcome, however, is most improbable without discipline, without parents establishing rules and expectations of behavior, and enforcing them—with punishment—if their children refuse to accept these boundaries. Such an outcome is also most improbable without *proper* punishment. As seen in the cases of millions of children throughout the world, *any* punishment does not equal *effective* punishment. Even though it might make some people sick, the truth is that adults who have been punished with the "rod of reproof" by their parents in a decent and respectful manner when they were children, *can* thank their parents. They have something to be thankful for, as their parents have made the *right* choices for their children.

The Promise of an Eternal Life

The Bible is very clear about what is to be expected from children. In Deuteronomy 5:16 it is stated, "Honor your father and your mother, as the Lord your God has commanded you. . . ." This command to children means that they should subject themselves to the authority of their parents—authority given to parents by God. A child should therefore respect his parents, obey them, and take their admonitions to heart (See Prov. 1:8, 13:1, and 20:20; Matt. 15:4, and Col. 3:20).

This command in Deuteronomy also holds a promise to children, because it continues to state, "so that you may live long and that it may go well with you in the land the Lord your God is giving you." This promise not only relates to the individual, but also to a civilization as a whole. The survival of a civilization is dependent on the maintenance of this command. This truth can be seen clearly in the history of previous civilizations—time and time again. In the early days of a civilization, this command is usually strictly *enforced*. As a civilization becomes older, more and more children of each new generation are *allowed* to refuse to submit themselves to the values and norms of older generations, with the result that the civilization gradually disintegrates and eventually dies.

The use of the two words *enforced* and *allowed* is intentional. As already stated, few children—if any—will submit themselves willingly to the authority of their parents, unless they have been *taught* to do so. As has been stated over and over in this book, there is nothing that any person knows, or can do, that he has not been taught. A child must therefore be *taught* to respect his parents, obey them, and take their admonitions to heart. And unless a child has learned to obey the command in Deuteronomy 5:16, he will not be able to submit himself to God's other commandments. If he is allowed to ignore a parent's admonition that lying is wrong, why would he obey Deuteronomy 5:20, —"You shall not give false testimony against your neighbor?"

The object of the command "Honor your father and your mother" is therefore not to establish an empty master-servant relationship. It serves to establish an authoritative relationship in which a more experienced person—one who presumably already *knows* right from wrong—can teach a younger person to *distinguish* right from wrong.

As already stated in the previous chapter, example and instruction are important tools in teaching a child to honor his parents. But, as also stated, due to his sinful nature, a child *will* trespass this command. Unless he is an angel and not a child, chances are that he might call his father or mother a "big stinker," throw a tantrum in a shopping center, disobey them, and lie in their faces.

When a parent is confronted with a child who is disobedient, disrespectful, or who oversteps the boundaries that have been taught to him by means of example and instruction, a parent has no choice but to take action. Proverbs 13:24 is quite clear about the action that needs to be taken: "He who spares the rod hates his son, but he who loves him is careful to discipline him."

As already stated, an objection to corporal punishment that is frequently raised by psychology and psychiatry is that it causes children to be violent or aggressive. The parent who spanks his child—according to psychology—punishes aggression with aggression and therefore sets an example of aggression to the child. If we study Proverbs 13:24, however, it is clear that spanking is not aggression at all—or, at least, it is not supposed to be—but love. Parents, however, have been grossly misled by the foolishness of psychology over the past few decades. The result is that many parents who still find corporal punishment acceptable view it as a last resort. If all else has failed, they will resort to corporal punishment, after having talked and talked, nagged, scolded, screamed, threatened, and applied other psychological methods of punishments such as "time-out."

The problem about this kind of behavior, which has become commonplace in our homes, is that children are no longer taught to listen. Remember that no human being can do anything that he has not been taught to do. A parent who repeats requests and commands over and over and over is conditioning his child that the noise emerging from an adult's mouth is nothing but hot air; just wait, it will come again. The same thing happens when a person lives near a railroad. Before long he learns to shut himself off so that he does not hear the noise any more.

Another problem is that no parent can repeat an instruction in the same tone of voice as the first time. A few decibels are added to each repetition and before long the parent is screaming and yelling at his child, thereby lashing the child with his *tongue*—the cruelest instrument that can possibly be used to hit the child. If, eventually, the confrontation between parent and child does end in corporal punishment, it is always accompanied by anger. Even parents who say that they are opposed to corporal punishment are sometimes inclined to strike their children—sometimes on just any part of their bodies—when driven to the point of exasperation. It is to things like these—hitting the child with the tongue, hitting in anger—that are referred in Proverbs 13:24 when it is stated: "He who spares the rod *hates* his son." The inevitable shouting and screaming which follows when requests and commands are repeated, as well as the uncontrollable lashing which might follow, cannot be experienced by the child as anything other than hatred—and it should be logical to any person that hatred and aggression are blood-brothers. If corporal punishment does lead to violence and aggression as psychology claims, *this* is the reason why. By depriving parents of the possibility of correcting their children's behavior with a spanking early in the conflict while a parent's emotions are still under control, they have driven love out of the home, and brought in hatred.

Apart from the fact that its abolition serves the hidden agendas of many of their adherents, there is also another reason why psychology and psychiatry continue to maintain that corporal punishment is unacceptable. This is that they have not been able to escape from the totally misplaced idea that John Locke proclaimed more than three centuries ago. According to Locke, the child is a *tabula rasa*—a clean slate on which anything may be written. This implies that the child enters this world as an innocent being and that the responsibility of society is to write the correct inscriptions on this clean slate. If the child errs later in life, it is because the wrong inscriptions were made.

The Bible, on the contrary, states very clearly that a child is not innocent, but that he comes into the world as an inherently sinful being. "Even from birth the wicked go astray; from the womb they are wayward and speak lies," the psalmist states in Psalms 58:3. Fortunately, a child does not enter the world only with wickedness in his heart, but also with a beautiful and noble possibility. This possibility, however, will remain a mere possibility, and can only be turned into a reality through the hard work of loving parents. Initially the wickedness in the child's heart is also just a mere possibility. This wicked possibility needs no encouragement to become a reality, however. In fact, unless it is forcibly suppressed, even the sweetest-looking baby will soon turn into a veritable little monster. The Bible leaves no uncertainty as to the *only* method through which this wicked possibility needs to be suppressed: "Folly is bound up in the heart of a child, but the rod of discipline will drive it far from him," states Proverbs 22:15. Every now and then, therefore, the parent is granted an opportunity to drive some of this folly from the child's heart. If he does this often enough (the regularity will differ from child to child), and well enough (this also depends on the individual child), the child will eventually lead a decent and virtuous life as an adult, and not be a murderer, rapist, thief, drug addict or alcoholic. Nobody can deny that people who become criminals, or drug addicts, or alcoholics, or something similar, lead very unhappy lives. The parent who chastises his child according to biblical criteria, wishes for his child to have the same good life that he as parent enjoys—or even better. Therefore, Proverbs 13:24 states, "but he who *loves* him is careful to discipline him." It is an act of love to spank a child, and not an act of aggression, as is wrongly and foolishly declared by psychology. It protects the child from the extreme unhappiness of life as a murderer, rapist, thief, drug addict, or alcoholic.

No wonder then that in connection with this there is a very clear and direct instruction in the Bible to parents. In Proverbs 23:13 it is stated clearly and to the point: "Do not withhold discipline from a child. . . ." Of course, there are people who try to rationalize this verse by arguing that other psychological methods of discipline are equally effective. But no, it is immediately clarified *exactly* what is meant by "discipline." This verse continues by stating, "if you punish him with the rod. . . ." This leaves no room for dispute whether such ridiculous and outlandish methods of punishment as taking away privileges or "time-out" may perhaps be referred to here.

This biblical command is followed by a promise. Proverbs 23:13 states, "Do not withhold discipline from a child; if you punish him with the rod, *he will not die.*"

What a remarkable promise, one that is of far greater significance than the promise that is made to the child in Deuteronomy. The promise in Deuteronomy concerns the child's earthly life, but this promise in Proverbs suggests that the responsibility of creating the possibility of an eternal life for a child is in the hands of his parent. It makes one shudder if one realizes just *how great* the responsibility is that rests on the shoulders of a parent. The following verse, Proverbs 23:14, removes all doubt that may still have lingered in the mind concerning this: "Punish him with the rod and save his soul from death."

We know that many theologians would not agree with us on this point, with the argument that our salvation is no longer dependent on the law, but on *grace* (Eph. 2:8). Grace, however, is not *a license to sin.* As Jesus said in Matthew 5:17-20:

> Do not think that I have come to abolish the Law or the Prophets; I have not come to abolish them but to fulfil them. (18) I tell you the truth, until heaven and earth disappear, not the smallest letter, not the least stroke of a pen, will by any means disappear from the Law until everything is accomplished. (19) Anyone who breaks one of the least of these commandments and teaches others to do the same will be called least in the kingdom of heaven, but whoever practices and teaches these commands will be called great in the kingdom of heaven. (20) For I tell you that unless your righteousness surpasses that of the Pharisees and the teachers of the law, you will certainly not enter the kingdom of heaven.

The only hope and help for our threatened children today is for us parents to return to the biblical blueprint, to honor and obey God, to teach His moral laws to our children and also live them to the full. Because he who does not only say "Lord, Lord," but also puts His words into practice after hearing them,

> . . . is like a man building a house, who dug down deep and laid the foundation on rock. When a flood came, the torrent struck that house but could not shake it, because it was well built. But he who hears my words and does not put them into practice is like a man who built a house on ground without a foundation. The moment the torrent struck that house, it collapsed and its destruction was complete. (Luke 6:46-49)

Notes

1. Detzer, K., "Whiting doesn't spare the rod: An unusual judge shows youthful offenders that 'there is no glamour in trouble,'" *Reader's Digest,* May 1963, in *World Corporal Punishment Research Website,* www.corpun.com.

2. *Beeld,* 10 September 1996.

3. "Don't spare the rod in disciplining children," *Atlanta Inquirer,* 11 January 1997, in *World Corporal Punishment Research Website.*

4. Miller, R., "What happened to discipline?" *Milwaukee Journal Sentinel,* 29 November 1998, in *World Corporal Punishment Research Website.*

5. Chigbo, O., "Antispanking activists should take a time-out," 1998, in *World Corporal Punishment Research Website.*

6. Farrell, C., *World Corporal Punishment Research Website,* www.corpun.com

7. Chigbo, "Antispanking activists should take a time-out."

8. "Britons favour canings in schools: Polls," *Straits Times,* 4 November 1996, in *World Corporal Punishment Research Website.*

9. Glover, S., "Can boys be beaten?" *Daily Telegraph,* 1 November 1996.

10. Ibid.

11. "Britons favour canings in schools: Polls," *Straits Times.*

12. "Students should be caned," *Agence France-Presse,* 30 December 1997.

13. "City schools turning into battlefields," *Cape Argus,* 24 April 1997.

14. Ngcai, S., "Sparing the cane is spoiling the child," *Cape Argus,* 6 June 1997.

15. Stensrud, R., & Burnett, D., "While Americans debate classroom discipline, there's not much debate in Japan," *US Magazine,* 14 June 1977, in *World Corporal Punishment Research Website.*

16. Kirkwood, R. C., "Best friends worst parents," *The Ottawa Sun,* 26 January 1999, 15.

17. Ibid.

18. Chigbo, "Antispanking activists should take a time-out."

19. Ibid.

20. "Heal thyself," *Hoaxes and Deceptions* (Alexandria, Virginia: Time-Life Books), 131-133.

13.

The Other Side of the Coin

All human beings have a need for acceptance that can only be satisfied through *love*. Evidence of this fact was observed as early as the thirteenth century, when Frederick II conducted an experiment with a number of infants. He wanted to determine what the original language was, and hoped that these children would start speaking it if they never had the opportunity to hear a word in any language. To accomplish this dubious research project, he assigned foster mothers to bathe and suckle the babies, but forbade them to fondle, pet, or talk to their charges. The experiment failed because all the children died.[1] The historian Salimbene wrote of Frederick's research subjects in 1248, "They could not live without petting."

Strangely, this rather cruel experiment of Frederick II did not cause the idea of parental indifference towards children to die out. No wonder then that Carver stated, "the one thing man has learned from history is that he doesn't learn anything from history."[2] Behaviorist John B. Watson certainly did not learn anything from Frederick II's horrible mistake, because he advised mothers not to hug and kiss their children, and never to let them sit on their laps. Watson was particularly afraid of too close a relationship between mother and child, for he recommended that mothers should sometimes leave their infants for some weeks so that they would not become dependent on them.[3] How important it is for a child to be close to his parents, however, came to light during World War II in Britain. With a view to the terrible air raids, a large number of children were carted from London to the country. There they were cared for in safety, but they deteriorated physically and emotionally to such an extent that they had to be brought back.[4]

More recently, Gary and Anne Marie Ezzo earned fame for a child-rearing program that they developed through their church in the suburbs of Los Angeles. Their book, *On Becoming Babywise*, published by their family-run company Growing Families International, is a best-seller. At least one million babies are apparently being raised according to their philosophy.[5] In their program the Ezzos advocate strict parental discipline, with which we agree in principle. It seems, however, that the *future* of the child is not the focus of the discipline, but the ease and comfort of the parent. This implies that it is a parent-centered educational philosophy, rather than a child-centered one. To our minds, it is doubtful whether a style of education that is not primarily for the benefit of the child can be regarded as education at all.

The Ezzos warn that babies can be spoiled through too much cuddling, and that a mother who feeds her baby girl on demand is "in bondage to her daughter's unpredictability." Quoting freely from the Bible, they say babies should be left to cry because "God did not intervene when His Son cried out on the cross."[6] The mistake they are making here is one that is very common in psychology: they overlook that there is a radical difference between a child and an adult. Jesus was not a child when He cried out on the cross, so this has no relevance to a baby's crying.

This practice of ignoring babies, who cry to be fed, is becoming increasingly popular with parents exasperated by screaming infants and sleepless nights. In most cases this practice is successful in the short term, because most babies soon learn to sleep through the night. Reports of babies raised in accordance with the Ezzos' methods being admitted to casualty units, dangerously dehydrated and underweight, however, cause one to sincerely question its wisdom.[7] And, Margaret Mead, an ethnologist, described an interesting phenomenon which indicates that this practice, even though it might have good results in many cases in the short term, might have adverse effects in the long term.

Mead tells about a tribe who inhabits two different sections of a South Sea island. The island is divided by an impassable mountain range, so that there can be no contact between the inhabitants of the two territories. The members of the two groups look alike, speak the same language, have the same religion, beliefs, and customs, and eat the same kind of food. Yet, the people on the one side of the island are extremely friendly and gentle, while the inhabitants of the other side of the mountain are quick-tempered, suspicious, and aggressive. In her investigation Dr. Mead could find only *one* cause for this strange phenomenon. The mothers of the friendly tribe are always in the presence of their babies. The moment the baby awakes, he is picked up and caressed and the mother feeds him before he is too hungry. The mothers on the other side of the mountain have a different approach. They leave their infants to cry until they are completely out of breath before they pick them up. Then the baby not only suckles from his mother's breast—he is so enraged that he, so to speak, revenges himself on his mother who has neglected him. This attitude of rage that accompanies the feeding time, she claims, becomes a permanent part of the child's temper.[8]

In another publication, *Preparing for Parenting*, the Ezzos scorn the significance of bonding with one's baby soon after birth. "In biblical times," they maintain, "a new mother did not lounge around in her bathrobe for weeks on end trying to establish a bond with her child."[9]

This, of course, is not true. In biblical times the issue of child rearing was not taken lightly. In 1 Samuel 1:21 and further we read that Hannah did not want to go up with her family to the annual sacrifice to the Lord, but first wanted to wean her son. In biblical times, a child was weaned quite late, at the age of two or three.

The reason why bonding between mother and child, but also between father and child, is so important, is for the sake of *identification*, a need of the child meaning *making-to-be-the-same*, an attitude of *I-want-to-be-like-you*.

A Compass for His Life

Identification can be compared to a traveler who wants to travel from one place to another, but does not know the way. He therefore needs a map. A child who enters this world is in exactly the same situation. He also has a destination—he must become a grown-up man or grown-up woman—but he does not know how to get there. Consequently, he needs a "map" in the form of a grown-up person, somebody who has already traveled along this route and who therefore can lead him to adulthood.

Parents are the primary educators of their children, and therefore the most important persons with whom their children will identify themselves. Children identify with their parents' daily customs and habits, careers and work, social life, religion and beliefs, attitudes, behavioral codes, and their values and norms. When a child is still at the beginning of his journey to adulthood, either Dad or Mom can serve equally well as identification figures. As the child gets closer to his final destination, however, more specific identification is required. At some point a boy will have a strong need to identify with his father, while a daughter would want to identify with her mother. This does not imply that the parent of the opposite sex is no longer important. As a matter of fact, this parent presents the image of the opposite sex to the child and the parents' relationship with each other teaches the child how a man and a woman are supposed to behave towards one another.

When a parent is a poor identification figure, or has a poor relationship with his child, several unfavorable outcomes may follow. A daughter, for example, who has an unpleasant father, can become suspicious towards or afraid of all men. On the other hand, if the relationship with the parent of the same sex is poor, the child may identify with the parent of the opposite sex, with homosexuality as a possible outcome. Martin Hallett, director and counselor at True Freedom Trust, has found that the majority of male homosexuals counseled identified very strongly with this lack of intimate bonding with the father or any other male role model.[10] Sara Lawton, a Christian counselor specializing in lesbianism and sex abuse, sees the root of female homosexuality as an unmet need for mother love. The heterosexual identity is not established and the child later suffers from a lack of confidence and fear of failure in heterosexual contacts. He or she tries to meet this unmet need by having sexual relationships with persons of the same sex.[11]

As stated above, a child's parents are the first and most important figures with whom a child will identify. As the child grows older, he also starts to identify with other people. When he goes to school, his loyalty can seemingly be transferred from his mother to his teacher. In due course, a boy might identify with a sports hero, while a girl might identify with a model or an actress. Of course, this happens only *after* he or she has identified with some comic-strip character, such as *Batman* (we admit that we are perhaps not up to date with the latest fads).

At a certain stage the need for identification with the parent is shifted to his or her peer group. The phase of puberty has dawned, and *I-want-to-be-like-you* makes room for *I-want-to-be-myself.* In most cases this is a difficult phase, both for parent and child. In the case of a child who is accustomed to having everything his own way, this phase is bound to be a nightmare.

In his desire to attain independence, the teenager often feels that he may not be like his parents, and is often overcritical of his "old-fashioned" parents. The search for his own identity causes great uncertainty, and now he looks for help and safety within his peer group. This need for acceptance with his friends is so great that he wants to prove this acceptance visibly and actively. The teenagers' mode of dress is therefore also a type of uniform. It is the "in" thing to dress, speak, and act in a certain way, to use certain expressions, and to listen to certain music.

The dark side of a person's need for identification is the fear of being rejected. Especially in the teenage years, during which time the young person is painfully aware of his changing body, which causes him to feel insecure even more, the fear of being rejected comes strongly to the fore. He will then sacrifice quite a lot not to be rejected. Mindful of the statistics previously recorded that drug abuse, sexual promiscuity, and delinquency are also the "in" things today, it is quite understandable that many parents dread their children's teenage years long before they have started.

The light at the end of this tunnel is that a child's identification with strangers and his peer group occurs only *after* the stage of identification with his parents. Parents thus have the opportunity, while their children are still young and impressionable, to teach *real* values to their children by means of *example, instruction,* and *punishment.* Even if the teenager does not follow the *person* of the parent any longer, the *values* his parents have taught him remain with him and can serve as a *compass* for his life.[12]

This compass is an aid according to which not only the fragile teenager, but also the later adult, can make choices. Man's life consists of a succession of choices. In every action, in everything any person says or does, he is continually contemplating various possibilities. To make the right choice he is dependent on a values system, more specifically a *hierarchy of values.* Imagine, for example, a situation where heavy peer pressure is put on a child to use drugs. If he already has a more or less fixed value system at his disposal, he will be *capable* of making a *responsible* choice between the value that friendship is important and the value that his body is a temple of God. If he chooses the former, he also chooses the consequence of drug abuse, which, in effect, is suicide—not so dramatically as jumping from a building, but just as final. If he chooses the latter, he also chooses the possibility—or certainty—of being rejected.

Therefore, a child who undertakes his journey to adulthood without a fixed values system and hierarchy of values, is as vulnerable as a traveler without a map or compass. Without a compass to help him choose between right and wrong, he will easily crumble under peer pressure. He will be forced to make a choice, but his choice will in all probability be between cocaine, heroin, LSD, or Ecstacy.

One could easily feel totally overwhelmed by the responsibility attached to parenthood, once one begins to really understand the enormity of this responsibility. Unfortunately, this responsibility does not yet end when a child reaches puberty. Although it is true that a teenager has an increasing need for freedom, and it should also increasingly be given to him, the parent still has to lead the child to exercise this freedom with responsibility. As stated earlier, freedom does not imply the absence of limits. One should also not forget that a teenager is still human, and therefore he is also fallible.

What Love *Is* and What It Is *Not*

While it is true that our modern world has various benefits, it has also greatly reduced the time parents have available to spend with their children. Previously, mothers could afford to stay at home. Today, most are compelled to work to make ends meet. This has led to fewer opportunities for communication between mother and child. Most fathers have also, in our modern world, become so involved in the rat race that they have withdrawn from the education of their children, leaving whatever involvement is still left between parents and children to their spouses. Another characteristic of our times that has a distressing effect on many children is the disintegration of the family unit. An increasing number of children are raised in single-parent families. Single parenthood is twice as demanding as a normal family—there isn't anybody to share our everyday duties— with the result that there is even less time left for children.

Within these realities, it is, however, essential that we examine our priorities. A child will not know that we accept and love him unless we *make* time to talk to him and also to *listen* to him. Except for his need for communication, he also needs to be kissed, cuddled and hugged (although most teenagers will probably take offense if you do this *in front of* their friends). A child does not only have a need to hear that we love him, but he needs to feel it as well. A child can be spoiled by an abundance of materialistic goods and by always getting his way, but a profusion of verbal and physical expressions of love will never spoil a child.

Parents who do not spend enough time with their children— simply because they do not *make* time—often feel guilty and try to compensate for this lack of time by lavishing pocket money and gifts on their children. However, as the well-known late South African educationist Pistorius remarked, "The child needs our presence, not our presents."[13] In such a case the parent's acceptance of the child, which he believes is proven by the gifts, is no more than pretense: the money and gifts are actually meant to buy peace of mind for the parent. Children quickly see through this and learn how to exploit the situation and to manipulate the parent to give more and more and more. Tragically, however, money and gifts cannot buy love. Therefore, children who grow up under such circumstances, almost invariably become some of the most wretched souls on earth. Human beings can sometimes survive without love, but it is scarcely a tolerable existence.

In other cases, there are parents who try to compensate with materialistic goods for a *lack of interest.* Children, however, are not that easily deceived. Very often, a child's misbehavior is a misplaced effort to force the parent to accept him and give him attention.

The other extreme of the "absent parent syndrome" is the parent who suffers from a "cotton ball syndrome." One often finds that parents who had to wait very long for their first child, or had to go through the trauma of a child with a severe illness, or gave birth to a child with a physical or mental handicap, wrap their child in cotton balls. They overprotect the child and do literally everything for him. It is easy to have understanding for such parents. When you love your children so much that you get a lump in your throat every time you think of them, it is hard not to overprotect them, let alone after they had to go through a trauma of some sort. But true love, unfortunately, has to be tough sometimes. The consequence of overprotection (excluding overprotection as far as their physical safety is concerned) is that the child gets so used to everything being done for him that he never learns to exert himself and never acquires any sense of responsibility. Very often these overprotected children are also allowed to do as they please, as the parents are often afraid that the child would not love them if they set limits to his behavior. Nothing, however, is further from the truth. Love and discipline are like two sides of the same coin. One side cannot exist without the other. One can also compare it to a plant that needs *both* sunshine and water to grow. A child who receives only discipline, but no love, is like a plant who receives water, but no sunshine. It will wither and die. The child, on the other hand, who receives only love, but no discipline, is like a plant that receives only sunshine, but no water.

It will also wither and die.

The child who is raised without adequate discipline very often becomes an outcast. He doesn't cooperate in the classroom, with the result that his teachers don't approve of him. He is also unpopular with his peers because he often makes a nuisance of himself, not awaiting his turn, but butting into their games. The result is that not only is his need for security not being responded to, but also his need for acceptance. This causes his behavior to deteriorate even further. The child is caught in a vicious circle, which makes it easy to understand why symptoms like low self-esteem and depression are often associated with a behavior disorder.

The most important persons, however, from whom the child needs love, is from his parents. Yes, there are parents who do not love their children. There are millions of children who are subjected to physical, emotional, and sexual abuse, who are left with scars for the rest of their lives. Abuse and love will never go hand in hand. But neither will passivity and love. Love requires action. If our children feel lonely, they need our companionship. When they are afraid, they need the safety of our embrace. If they are happy, they need to share their laughter and cheerfulness with us. When they ask *Who loves me?* we need to take them into our arms and tell them how much we care. But if they are defiant and ask *Who is in charge?* we need to answer with discipline and teach them how to control their impulses and urges.

The Gold of Which the Coin Is Made

Although we have mentioned the present-day practice of scolding and screaming at children in the previous chapter, the effect on children is so destructive that we have to warn against this practice once again. When used in a decent and proper manner, the "rod of reproof" cannot do our children any harm. It can only do them good. Lashing a child with a tongue, however, can scar him for life.

Every person has a need for *dignity*, a striving for acknowledgment, appreciation, and a feeling of importance. This need can only be satisfied through *respect*. When this need is taken care of, a person experiences a feeling of self-confidence. He feels that he is useful, valuable, and even necessary. If this need is neglected, it leads to feelings of inferiority. If we scold and scream at our children, we are conveying the message that we do not respect them. Therefore we cannot expect of them to respect us in return.

If love and discipline are like two sides of the same coin, respect is the gold of which the coin is made. With it, the coin is priceless. Without it, there is no gold and the coin is worthless.

Notes

1. Dobson, J., *Dare to Discipline* (Toronto: Bantam Books, 1977), 33.

2. Blatt, B., "Lessons from history," *Journal of Learning Disabilities*, vol. 18(1), 1985, 18.

3. Watson, J. B., & Watson, R., *Psychological Care of Infant and Child* (London: Allen and Unwin, 1928).

4. Pistorius, P., *Kind in Krisis* (Human & Rousseau: Cape Town, 1981), 31.

5. Langton, J., "Spock challenged by the philosophy of a good smack," *Sunday Times*, 1 March 1998, 12.

6. Ibid.

7. Ibid.

8. Pistorius, *Kind in Krisis*, 42-43.

9. Langton, "Spock challenged by the philosophy of a good smack."

10. Hallet, M., *Nucleus*, January 1994.

11. Lawton, S., "Lecture 8 in signposts to wholeness," *True Freedom Trust*, 1994.

12. Pistorius, *Kind in Krisis*, 32.

13. Ibid., 64.

14.

The Keys to the Kingdom

deer momee and dadee

I bo not wont to go to shool eny more becouse the children ar lafing at me I canot reed pleese help me

your sun david

David is not a dunce. In fact, according to the evaluations of a few professionals, he is rather intelligent. Yet he certainly has a problem, and he shares his problem with millions of other children and adults. David, according to these professionals, is dyslexic.

The word "dyslexia" comes from the Greek, meaning "difficulty with words or language." Perhaps the simplest modern definition of dyslexia is that it is a difficulty in learning to read and write—particularly in learning to spell correctly and to express one's thoughts on paper.[1]

Dyslexia, as ADHD, is a subject that belongs to the study field of learning disabilities (LD). Although a multitude of other disabilities are found within the LD field, a reading disability—or dyslexia—is the most common. Estimates of learning-disabled students having dyslexia vary between 70 and 85 percent. Some experts are of the opinion that this percentage is even higher, so much so that labeling a child as learning disabled is understood to include a reading disability.[2] Whatever the exact figure might be, the importance of reading in the learning situation is as plain as a pikestaff. Dewey and his followers would of course oppose this view. But those who have not fallen under his spell still regard reading as the most important skill which a child must acquire at school,[3] because one must learn to read in order to be able to read to learn.[4] The implication of this is that the child who is a poor reader will usually also be a poor learner.

In our modern society where academic achievement is regarded as of great importance, persistent learning failure leads to anguish, embarrassment and frustration. Children are often treated like dunces by their teachers and mocked by their classmates. A learning disability certainly has a traumatic effect on a child's self-esteem. "He or she could be an Einstein," remarked British actress Susan Hampshire, who is dyslexic, "but if you don't read by your sixth birthday, who cares about your potential! Underachieving at school can be a major blow to the confidence and leave its scars for the rest of your life."[5]

Literacy is also the key to *employment,* and what awaits the LD child outside the school gates is probably nothing but a hopeless future:

> Many LD young adults are employed in jobs that offer little personal satisfaction or opportunity for advancement. Many others are not finding employment at all. Many are unsuccessful in their pursuit of further training . . . Many LD young adults have major academic, social and vocational needs that make it hard for them to make friends, live independent lives, and feel good about themselves.[6]

The above quotations suggest that human beings, besides other needs, also have an intellectual need—the need to *know.* The method through which this need is satisfied, of course, is by *learning.*

ADHD goes hand in hand with intellectual problems like reading, spelling, and writing "disabilities," poor academic performance and progress, and even a low intelligence. The future happiness and success of children with ADHD is thereby put in the balance. This means that the issue of learning, and especially reading, cannot be omitted in any discussion of ADHD. As Richardson stated so succinctly, "Literacy gives us the keys to knowledge and wisdom—the keys to the Kingdom. . . . [Shouldn't we] see that those keys are given to every child?"[7]

Getting help for these children's intellectual problems, however, seems to be easier said than done. If one studies the literature on the results achieved in the LD field with conventional intervention programs, one soon discovers that these results have been deplorable since the discovery of learning disabilities in the 1960s, and have not improved since.

Very soon after the LD notion took off, remedial programs of different types were under way, ranging from small one-enthusiastic-teacher size programs to large, nationally funded ones. However, a disappointing shock came to many special educators when the President's Report to Congress, reported by Nixon in 1970 in *American Education,* stated its findings. After spending one billion dollars on compensatory education, mainly for reading skills, only 19 percent of children improved their reading significantly, 15 percent fell behind more than expected, and more than two-thirds of the children remained unaffected. That is, they continued to fall behind.[8]

After reviewing a set of long-term studies, Spreen concluded in 1982, "most children who are referred for a learning or reading disability do not catch up. In fact, their disability is likely to become worse in time. In addition, remedial instruction has not been shown to improve the prognosis of these children."[9] Similarly, citing the results of a longitudinal study, Bashir and Scavuzzo stated in 1992, "there is little evidence of 'catch-up' of academic abilities."[10] Zigmond and Thornton noted, "Despite concerted efforts at early intervention and remedial teaching, learning disabilities are pervasive and persistent,"[11] and Coles, another authority in the field, concurs:

> A number of the children have been helped. . . . Most of them, however, have been helped very little. They enjoy minimal academic success throughout their school years, and as learning failure deepens, so does frustration, disappointment, and insecurity. Their reading and other learning problems are likely to continue into adulthood, with destructive effects on their feelings of self-worth, personal relationships, and job opportunities and performance.[12]

There can be only two explanations for this inability of experts to assist the reading disabled. The first explanation may be that they are trying to solve an unsolvable problem. Statements such as "learning disabilities are usually incurable,"[13] "the learning weakness will always remain,"[14] and "dyslexia is like alcoholism . . . it can never be cured"[15] are often found in the literature. Other statements are even more dooming. According to Stanovich, not only do poor readers retain their low position in the achievement hierarchy, but they actually become more discrepant from good readers over time; hence the "poor get poorer and rich get richer" allusion.[16]

The only other explanation for the deplorable results obtained in the LD field is that reading disabilities are in fact curable, but the experts in the field are still groping in the dark to find a cure. As already mentioned, a solution to most problems is dependent on knowing the *cause* or causes of that problem. To illustrate the present state of affairs on this point, we quote Hallahan, Kauffman, and Lloyd, "But what actually is *known* about why children are learning disabled? The answer to this question is 'very little!' "[17]

If "very little" is *known* about why children are learning disabled, it implies that whatever is regarded as the cause or causes of this problem may be based on no more than guesswork. The causes are *presumed* and as we all know, presumptions can easily be wrong.

As in the case of ADHD, the popular explanation—LD experts refer to this explanation as a *fact*—for a learning or reading disability is that there is something wrong inside the child's brain. In accordance with this view, learning is a neurological process which takes place inside the brain. On these grounds it is supposed that the child who struggles to read or learn must have a neurological dysfunction. Yet, as in the case of ADHD, this explanation is nothing but a mere myth. In the most comprehensive study of this type, the so-called National Collaborative Perinatal Project, the relationship between neurological signs and learning disabilities in 7-year-olds could account for only 1 percent of the learning problems.[18] And in another study, children with the most "neurological signs" actually had the fewest learning problems.[19]

It should be noted that, even *if* neurological differences were to be found between LD and non-LD students, the question still remains which of the two, the neurological dysfunction or the reading disability, is the *cause* and which one is the *effect?* It is well-known that intellectual stimulation changes brain structure, and therefore neurological differences of a structural nature is not necessarily the cause of a learning or reading disability, but can also be the *effect.*

It seems that the present-day custom of attributing our children's learning and reading problems to biological explanations has had only one result, and that is to exempt educators from their responsibilities:

> The larger society is satisfied that it has an excuse, an expression to explain why somebody's kids don't learn. Similarly, many teachers are delighted with the rubric as an excuse for not teaching. Schools and homes, thus, have a catchall, with no pressure to change. For a headache, we take aspirin; for a difficulty in school, we take learning disabilities.[20]

Perhaps it has become time for LD specialists to seek alternative theories and avenues. As in the case of ADHD, this theory has so far done nothing but to destroy the lives of millions of children.

An Alternative Approach

Before we can start talking about learning, we first must define the *fundamental, species-specific characteristics*[21] of the species that we are studying—in this case man. These characteristics have so far been overlooked in the study of the learning and reading-disabled child. That is why this problem has remained a mystery for so long.

The sciences that traditionally occupy themselves with the study of the phenomenon of learning disabilities are mainly psychology, psychiatry, education, neurology, ophthalmology, and occupational therapy. None of these has as its aim the discovery of the fundamental, species-specific characteristics of the human being. This is the task of philosophy, specifically of philosophical anthropology. From whatever scientific perspective one wishes to study the LD child, one would therefore have to check with the philosopher first, to find out what fundamental characteristics of the human being might play a role in the situation.

The *first* of these species-specific characteristics that we need to take note of has already been discussed in detail. It is that there is *nothing that any human being knows, or can do, that he has not learned.* If one accepts this—that there is nothing that any human being can do that he has not learned to do—as a fundamental characteristic, it opens up new avenues of interpreting the problem of the child with a learning and reading disability. It implies that there is not necessarily anything wrong with a person who cannot do something. He is not necessarily *dyslexic* or *reading disabled.* He may simply not have learned to read properly yet—and any person can learn almost anything, provided that the other fundamental characteristics of the human being, that might play a role in human learning, are also taken into account.

The *second* important species-specific characteristic is that *human learning does not take place on a single level, but is a stratified process.* This characteristic is accepted worldwide as a didactic principle. The way in which the school system throughout the whole world is organized is an acknowledgment of this. One cannot send one's child to university first. He must start at the first class and then progress year after year to the higher levels of education. At the end of every year, the child is expected to provide proof—usually by passing an examination—that he has mastered a sufficient amount of the knowledge that had been presented to him during the year so that it will form a firm enough base on which to build the knowledge of the following year. If human learning had not been a stratified process, if it had taken place on a single level, this would have been unnecessary. It would then not have been important to start a child in first grade. It would have been possible for the child to enter school at any level, and to complete the school years in any order, for example ninth grade, fourth grade, then sixth grade, and so on.

Another simple and practical example is the fact that one has to learn to count before it becomes possible to learn to add and subtract. Suppose one tried to teach a child who had not yet learned to count to add and subtract. This would be quite impossible, and no amount of effort would ever succeed in teaching the child these skills. After months or years of fruitless effort one might also gain the impression that there had to be something wrong with the child's brain. However, if one first taught the child to count, it would become quite easy to teach him to add and subtract. This proves that counting is a skill that must be mastered before it becomes possible to learn to do calculations.

This means that there is a sequence that is to be observed when teaching people. Certain things have to be taught to them *first*, *before* it becomes possible to teach them other things.

This is a self-evident fact, yet, this very important principle of human learning, just as the other one that was mentioned earlier, is hardly noted in any of the present-day theories on learning. When considering the teaching of reading, for example, experts seem to overlook, and others do not seem to fully understand, how important it is that there are also certain skills and knowledge that a child must have acquired *before* it becomes possible for him to benefit from a course in reading.

Bartoli, who says that it "is the actual practice with the real task of reading that leads to more skillful reading," is only partially correct. "Of course," she adds, "any soccer, tennis, or basketball coach will tell you the same thing: if you want to get better, you have to play the game—not just practice skill drills."[22] Now, we know very little about tennis and basketball, but we do happen to know about soccer. The game of soccer consists of many elements—passing, control, shooting, dribbling, heading, and goal keeping. Before any child is expected to play well in a full-game situation, he must be able to pass, control, shoot, dribble, and head the ball. Unless these basic skills have been *automated,* the child will have two left feet on the soccer field.

The reading "game," just like the game of soccer, rests upon certain skills and until these skills have become automated, the child will have "two left eyes" in the reading situation. The important thing, of course, is to know *what* these skills are.

A "Pyramid of Repetition" Must Be Constructed

> Everyone wants education to be relevant. It is hard even to conceive why anyone would wish it to be irrelevant. Those who proclaim the need for "relevance" in education are fighting a straw man—and evading the crucial need to define what they mean by "relevance," and why that particular definition should prevail.[23]

Beginning in the 1960s, under the influence of Carl Rogers (see chapter nine), insistence on relevance became widespread. However, the particular kind of relevance sought was typically a relevance judged *in advance* by *students* who had not yet learned the particular things being judged, much less applied in practice in the real world. Relevance thus became a label for the general belief that the usefulness and meaningfulness of information or training could be determined *in advance*—by *students.*[24] Furthermore, the idea that instruction should equal entertainment replaced drilling and repetition, which became swear words in education.

Unfortunately, learning and reading disabilities will remain pervasive and persistent and there will always be little evidence of catch-up of academic abilities for as long as relevance—as it is presently defined—remains a sacred cow. If Bartoli is correct when she says, "Having to spend long periods of time on repetitive tasks is a sign that learning is not taking place—that this is not a productive learning situation,"[25] then adults will not pass a driver's license exam, actors won't be able to play their roles, sports fans will have no heroes, and there will be no musicians. In order to master any of these skills, repetition—and especially repetition of fragmented skills—is essential in the initial stages. In fact, top soccer players will confirm that in order to stay in shape, they still need to spend many hours on the practice of fragmented skills—passing, control, shooting, dribbling, and heading.

A full understanding of the *third* important species-specific characteristic of human learning, that *there must be enough repetition for a beginner learner,* will make it clear why the relevance notion has so greatly contributed to the deterioration of Western education.

A beginner learner must start by repeating a limited amount of material many times over and over. Gradually, less and less repetition will be necessary to master new skills and new knowledge. A "pyramid of repetition" must therefore be constructed. Evolutionist educators should take note, because this principle seems to apply even in the "teaching" of animals. The following example is quoted from the book *Nurtured by Love: A New Approach to Education*, authored by the late Japanese Shinichi Suzuki:

> In our Tokyo Shinagawa branch, headed by Mr. Miyazawa, was a little parakeet, the pet of tiny children who came there for their violin lessons. When Mr. and Mrs. Miyazawa bought the bird, the couple taught him to say in Japanese, "I am Peeko Miyazawa, I am Peeko Miyazawa." The bird, in his high-pitched voice, later said to the children what he had happened to hear: "Peeko is a good little bird, Peeko is a good little bird." According to Mr. Miyazawa, one must begin training a bird soon after birth. In the beginning one must have much perseverance, energy and patience. In order to make the parakeet speak, and develop his ability, it is necessary to repeat the same word over and over again. Just when we think it is useless, and despair, and want to give up, finally we are rewarded with some results.

> At first the name Peeko was repeated to the bird about fifty times daily; that made three thousand times in two months. Then, at last, the little bird began to say "Peeko" ...

> After teaching the bird to say, by repeating it three thousand times, "Peeko," "Miyazawa" was added. This time, after having heard "Peeko Miyazawa" daily for fifteen minutes, he could say it after only two hundred times."[26]

The point of this story is that much repetition was needed before Peeko could say the first word. Gradually, it became easier and easier, until eventually very little repetition was needed in order to add a new word or words. No doubt it is the same with man, as the following story also taken from Suzuki illustrates:

> Since 1949, our Mrs. Yano has been working with new educational methods for developing ability, and every day she trains the infants of the school to memorize and recite Issa's well-known haiku. [A haiku is a short Japanese poem, consisting only of three lines.] Children who at first could not

memorize one haiku after hearing it ten times were able to do so in the second term after three to four hearings, and in the third term only one hearing.[27]

This means that, if one systematically and regularly does repetition with a learner, it will gradually become possible for the learner to learn more and more with fewer and fewer repetitions. It is almost as if a "pyramid of repetition" has to be constructed first.

That this "pyramid of repetition" is relevant to learning situations beyond learning poems is seen in the learning of a first language. According to Beve Hornsby, it has been found that a child who is just beginning to talk must hear a word about five hundred times before it will become part of his active vocabulary (before he can say it).[28] Two years later, the same child will need only one to a few repetitions to learn to say a new word.

Without building this "pyramid of repetition" first, later learning will always be time consuming and prone to failure. Unfortunately educators have ignored this characteristic of human learning and have removed most of the repetitive work that used to form part of education for so long. With few exceptions, this change is seen as a step forward: "We overlooked what our common sense told us, which was that the poems that we had learned in school were useless for helping us to remember what we needed to buy at the supermarket."[29]

It seems that people, like Kronick, who regard this as a step forward, are wrong, because all over the world learning difficulties are escalating tremendously. One of the reasons for this increase in learning difficulties is that repetition (or drilling) has been dropped out of the school system. As Kronick said—the memorizing of poems would not help you to remember what to buy at the supermarket. What she does not realize—and many others, too—was that by reciting and repeating these poems over and over we were building this pyramid of repetition. Therefore, it was not useless at all!

In this respect, there are two very important factors that should be kept in mind: The first is that there is great individuality among different people, and even within the same person, in the amount of repetition required to learn something. The amount of repetition that is enough for one person may not necessarily be enough for another. The amount of repetition that a certain person requires in mastering a certain skill may not necessarily be enough to master another skill. Mrs. Butler might need ten lessons to master the skill of driving, Mrs. Brown might need twenty, Mrs. Lane thirty, and Mrs. Jones forty. But Mrs. Jones, who struggled to learn to drive, might need only ten lessons to become an expert in sewing. (Note that Mrs. Jones is not diagnosed as "driving disabled" because she needed forty lessons!)

The second important factor is that one should not lose sight of the stratified nature of learning. If a child has not yet mastered the skill of counting, 10,000 repetitions in adding and subtracting will not teach him to add and subtract. The child needs to learn how to count *first*, although he might need more repetitions to master this skill than other children might.

The *fourth* characteristic of human learning is that there must be opportunities for *application*. Even while a child is learning to master the fragmented elements of soccer, he can and should already be given opportunities to *apply* these skills in practice—in an actual game. In the same way, while learning to master the skills that form the basis of reading, a child can and should already be given opportunities to apply these skills in the act of reading.

An important point is that these four fundamental learning principles should be looked upon as a whole and should not be viewed in isolation. Any botanist will tell you the same thing: it is the whole of the amount of water, sunlight, and fertilizer that will cause a tree to bear large, juicy fruit. If you only water the tree six weeks after you have hoed the fertilizer into the ground, you are bound to return to a withered tree.

Notes

1. Hornsby, B., *Overcoming Dyslexia* (Johannesburg: Juta and Company Ltd., 1984), 9.

2. Coles, G., *The Learning Mystique* (New York: Pantheon Books, 1987), xii.

3. Blignaut, C. M., *'n Inleiding tot Leesonderrig* (Johannesburg: A. P. B., 1963).

4. Barkhuizen, B. P., *'n Psigologies-Pedagogiese Ondersoek van die Leesprobleem in Transvaalse Laerskole* (Unisa: Unpublished DEd thesis, 1963).

5. Hampshire, S., *Every Letter Counts. Winning in Life Despite Dyslexia*

(London: Corgi Books, 1991), 20.

6. Zigmond, N., & Thornton, H. S., "The future of learning disabilities," in K. A. Kavale (ed.), *Learning Disabilities: State of the Art and Practice* (Boston: College-Hill Press, 1988), 180-205.

7. Richardson, S., "Specific developmental dyslexia. Retrospective and prospective views," *Annals of Dyslexia,* vol. 39, 1989, 3-24.

8. Nixon, R., "Message on education reform," *American Education,* vol. 6(3), 1970.

9. Spreen, O., "Adult outcomes of reading disorders," in R. N. Malatesha & P. G. Aaron (eds.), *Reading Disorders: Varieties and Treatments* (New York: Academic Press, 1982).

10. Bashir, A. S., & Scavuzzo, A., "Children with language disorders: Natural history and academic success," *Journal of Learning Disabilities,* vol. 25, 1992, 53-65.

11. Zigmond & Thornton, "The future of learning disabilities."

12. Coles, G. S., "Excerpts from The Learning Mystique: A critical look at 'learning disabilities.' " *Journal of Learning Disabilities,* vol. 22(5), 1989, 267-277.

13. Winslow, R., "College for the learning disabled," *New York Times,* 22 February 1982.

14. Summers, J., "Special feature on learning disabilities," *Today's Education,* November-December 1977, 36-48.

15. Clark, M., & Gosnell, M., "Dealing with dyslexia," *Newsweek,* March 1982, 55-56.

16. Stanovich, K. E., "Matthew effects in reading: Some consequences of individual differences in the acquisition of literacy," *Reading Research Quarterly,* vol. 31, 1986, 360-406.

17. Hallahan, D. P., Kauffman, J., & Lloyd, J., *Introduction to Learning Disabilities* (Englewood Cliffs, NJ: Prentice Hall, 1985), 17.

18. Nichols, P., & Chen, T., *Minimal Brain Dysfunction: A Prospective Study* (Hillsdale, NJ: Lawrence Earlbaum, 1981).

19. Ingram, T. T. S., Mason, A. W., & Blackburn, I., "A retrospective study of 82 children with reading disability," *Developmental Medicine and Child Neurology,* vol. 12, 1970, 271-279.

20. Sabatino, D. A., "The house that Jack built," *Journal of Learning*

Disabilities, vol. 16(1), 1983, 26-27.

21. Schmidt, W. H. O., *Child Development: The Human, Cultural, and Educational Context* (New York: Harper & Row, 1973), xiii.

22. Bartoli, J. S., "An ecological response to Coles's interactivity alternative," *Journal of Learning Disabilities,* vol. 22(5), 1989, 292-297.

23. Sowell, T., *Inside American Education* (Englewood Cliffs: Julian Messner, 1993), 89.

24. Ibid.

25. Bartoli, "An ecological response to Coles's interactivity alternative."

26. Suzuki, S., *Nurtured by Love: A New Approach to Education* (New York: Exposition Press, 1969).

27. Ibid.

28. Hornsby, *Overcoming Dyslexia,* 43.

29. Kronick, D., New *Approaches to Learning Disabilities. Cognitive, Metacognitive and Holistic* (Philadelphia: Grune & Stratton, 1988).

15.

The Stratified Nature of Learning

Human learning, as we concluded, does not take place on a single level, but is a stratified process. There are certain skills that need to be mastered before any person can learn the skills of adding and subtracting, or the game of soccer. The same applies to reading. There are also skills and experiences that form the basis or *foundation* of reading and writing.

A foundation, according to the dictionary, is the "natural or prepared ground or base on which some structure rests." This means that "foundational skills of reading" would refer to skills that form the prepared ground or base on which the structure of reading rests. This would further mean that, unless this base has been prepared adequately, no effective reading can take place.

The Foundational Skills of Reading

The reading act is a unitary occurrence, meaning that the actions taking place while one is reading occur simultaneously. However, for the purpose of this discussion, these actions will be divided into steps, and a schematic diagram of the reading act is presented on the following page. It is advised that the reader refer to this diagram throughout the rest of this discussion.

Reception

Reading must be regarded as an act of communication. In any communication situation, two parties are involved, the sender of the message and the receiver of the message. The fact that physically only one party is present in the reading situation does not refute the statement that reading is an act of communication. There are indeed two parties involved, although the sender of the message is not physically present. The sender of the message is the author of the

ACT OF READING

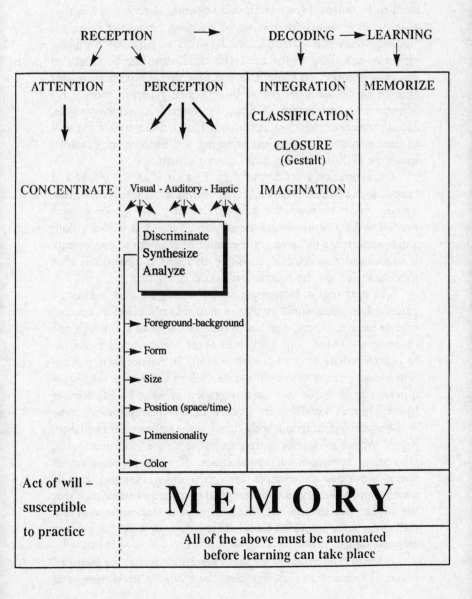

RECEPTION ⟶ DECODING ⟶ LEARNING

ATTENTION	PERCEPTION	INTEGRATION	MEMORIZE
		CLASSIFICATION	
		CLOSURE (Gestalt)	
CONCENTRATE	Visual - Auditory - Haptic	IMAGINATION	

Discriminate
Synthesize
Analyze

➤ Foreground-background

➤ Form

➤ Size

➤ Position (space/time)

➤ Dimensionality

➤ Color

Act of will –
susceptible
to practice

MEMORY

All of the above must be automated
before learning can take place

book that the reader is reading. He transferred his message to the reader or receiver of the message by means of symbols put on paper.

When reading, there are many factors involved in the reception of the message. The first of these is that the reader must *pay attention*. Paying attention is a body function, and therefore does not need to be taught. However, paying attention as such is a function that is quite useless for the act of learning, because it is only a fleeting occurrence. Attention usually shifts very quickly from one object or one thing to the next. The child must first be taught to *focus* his attention on something and to keep his attention on this something for some length of time. When a person focuses his attention for any length of time, we refer to it as *concentration*. Paying attention, therefore, is the body function that makes the skill of concentration possible, just as seeing and hearing, for example, make the skills of looking and listening possible.

Concentration rests on two legs. First, it is an *act of will* and cannot take place automatically. The will to focus attention on the message must be sustained in order to carry out all the actions needed to fully comprehend the message. Second, it is also a skill, and therefore has to be *taught*. Because the inability to concentrate is so prominent in ADHD, it will be discussed in more detail after this discussion on the foundational skills of reading.

The next step in receiving a written message is that it must be perceived. In other words, *perception* must take place. Before one can read or learn anything, one has to become aware of it through one of the senses. Usually one has to hear or see it. Subsequently, one has to *interpret* whatever one has seen or heard. In essence then, perception means interpretation. Of course, lack of experience may cause a person to be liable to misinterpretation of what he has seen or heard. Thus, in describing the phenomenon of perception, we come to the psychological truism aptly stated by the philosopher Immanuel Kant: "We see things not as they are but as we are." In other words, perception represents our apprehension of a present situation in terms of our past experiences. Perceptual ability, therefore, heavily depends upon the amount of perceptual practice and experience that the subject has already enjoyed. This implies that perception is a skill that can be improved tremendously through judicious practice and experience.

A further important point about perception is that the stratified nature of learning also applies here. Perception in itself consists of a large number of subskills that can all be automated. First, there are various ways of perceptualizing, namely visual, auditory, and haptic. The latter includes touch perception and kinesthetic perception. Because we read with our eyes, visual perception plays the most important role in the reading act, and will therefore be discussed at some length.

When a person is reading, visual *discrimination* must take place. All printed letters are set against a certain background. The most important difference between the letters and the background is that they differ in color. Obviously, the first discrimination will thus be in terms of *color*. The second discrimination is in terms of *foreground-background*. The particular letter, word, or sentence, that the reader is focused on is elevated to the level of foreground, whereas everything else within the field of vision of the reader (the rest of the page and the book, the desk on which the book is resting, the section of the floor and/or wall that is visible, etc.) is relegated to the background. Our Latin alphabet consists of twenty-six letters, including capital letters with a difference in size and sometimes in shape compared to their lower case counterparts. The letters all differ in *form* or *shape* and must be discriminated accordingly. Capital letters, used at the start of a sentence, sometimes look exactly the same as their lower case counterparts, and must therefore be discriminated mainly with regard to *size*. One also does not only read letters, but thoughts, all compiled from a conglomeration of words. A word is made up of a number of letters arranged in a particular sequence. The reader must therefore be able to discriminate the letters in terms of their *positions*. If a sketch or picture is included in the text, there must be discrimination of *dimensionality* as well.

After discriminating every letter with regard to color, foreground and background, form, size, and position, letters must be combined to understand the word. The reader must thus be able to perceive individual parts as a whole. In other words, he must be able to *synthesize*.

Although the ability to *analyze* (i.e. to perceive the whole in its individual parts) does play a role in reading, this ability is of the utmost importance in spelling. To be a good speller, one must be able to analyze.

The above events sound very complex, and indeed must be recognized as being just that. In reality, they take place all the time—at lightning speed—while a person is reading, but a good reader is unaware of these events because they have been automated. It can be compared to a Spaniard speaking Spanish while doing other things because his knowledge of the language has been automated through regular practice and usage. While speaking, he is not concentrating on grammar, word order, sentence structure, and things like that, but on the *contents* of what he wants to say. This is only possible because his language has become automatic.

Decoding

When a person attempts to speak a language that has not yet become automatic, he will necessarily have to divide his attention between the content of his message and the language itself. He will therefore speak haltingly and with great difficulty—just as a child, in whom the above-mentioned foundational skills of reading have not yet become automatic, also reads haltingly and with great difficulty. The poor reader is forced to apply all his concentration to the reception of the message, and therefore has "no concentration left" to decode the message.

The decoding of the message is a very important aspect of the reading act. Without being able to decode the message, the receiver cannot understand it. This explains why some children can "read" without understanding what they are reading.

Decoding implies that the reader is able to decipher the message; in other words, he is able to ascribe meaning to the written word. This becomes possible first by *integrating* the message that he is reading with his foreknowledge. If one reads something that cannot directly be connected to or tied in with knowledge that one already possesses, one cannot decode the message. Foreknowledge can be defined as the range of one's existing knowledge and past experiences. Everything one observes around one forms part of one's field of vision and meaning can be ascribed to it. Facts and experiences outside one's range of knowledge and past experiences do not make sense to one. If a person is reading a book that does not fall within his range of knowledge and experiences, he will not be able to decipher the contents of the message. Even here, therefore, the stratified nature of learning plays a role.

A decoding skill that is closely related to that of integration is *classification*. When a person sees a chair, although he may never have seen a chair exactly like this one, he will nevertheless immediately recognize it as a chair, because he is familiar with the *class* of objects we call "chair." This implies that, whenever a name is ascribed to an object, it is thereby put into a specific class of objects, or it is *classified*.

The Gestalt principle *closure* means that the mind is able to derive meaning from objects or pictures that are not perceived in full. I -m s-re th-t y-- w-ll b- -ble to und-rsta-d th-s s-ntence-, although more than 25 percent of the letters have been omitted. The mind is quite able to bridge the gaps that were left in the sentence. The idea of closure is, however, more than just seeing parts of a word and amplifying them. It also entails the amplification of the author's message. No author can put all his thoughts into words. This stresses the importance of foreknowledge. If it were possible for an author to put everything related to the subject he is dealing with on paper, foreknowledge would have been unnecessary. That, however, is impossible, as an author can at most present us with a very limited cross-section of reality and the reader must be able to expand this before comprehension becomes possible.

Lastly, *imagination* plays a role in decoding. While one is reading, one is also picturing the objects and ideas symbolized by the words. Should the author describe a beautiful landscape, one would actually picture this in the mind's eye. One does not merely see the words, one also "sees" the scene. This plays a very important role in decoding the message. Furthermore, by using one's imagination while reading, one's emotions can be addressed during the reading act.

Learning

Only after a person has decoded a message can learning take place. To learn, a person must be able to store something that he has perceived and decoded, so that he will be able to recall this information at a later stage. The ability to *recall to memory* or to remember, makes learning possible.

Memory is one of the foundational skills of learning which is of special importance in the so-called learning subjects at school or university, where information is presented to the learner, and it is expected that he be able to reproduce it as accurately as possible.

However, memory is a skill that is also of great importance to the reading act. For example, recognizing the shapes of the different letters comprising a particular word, is an act of memory. Every word also consists of letters in a particular sequence, and one has to remember what word is represented by the sequence of letters in question.

The Stratified Nature of Concentration

Concentration is foundational not only to reading, but to all other forms of learning. Without the ability to concentrate, learning cannot take place effectively.

As mentioned before, concentration rests on two legs. First, it is an *act of will* and cannot take place automatically. The *will* to focus attention in any learning situation must be sustained before effective learning can take place. Second, it is also a skill, and therefore has to be *taught*.

One often finds that children with so-called ADHD can concentrate very effectively in activities that are novel in some way, or in activities which they find enjoyable, such as playing computer games or watching TV. In fact, they can often do this for hours on end. Their inability to focus their attention is often related to school or schoolwork only. They cannot sit still, they fidget, swing their legs, play with their stationery, stare out through the window, annoy other children, and will sometimes even get up from their seats and walk around in the classroom. Homework sessions are often a nightmare, accompanied by tears or outbursts.

The cause of this phenomenon is not that some mysterious brain dysfunction "kicks in" the moment when a child is confronted by schoolwork, and "kicks out" when he starts playing video games. This behavior is simply the visible signs of a child who is not receptive for learning on an *emotional* level. *Before* a child can be receptive for learning on an intellectual level, he must be receptive on an emotional level. In other words, before one can teach a child the skill of concentration (i.e., *how* to concentrate), or before he can be taught anything else effectively, he must be *willing* to concentrate or focus his attention. In effect, he must be willing to *learn*.

How does one make a child willing to learn? The answer to this question should seem hackneyed by now. He must be *taught*. Although no human being can survive properly in our world without learning, willingness or eagerness to learn is not an innate human quality. As in the case of friendliness, thankfulness, honesty, unselfishness, and a respect for authority, willingness, or eagerness to learn is a quality that can only be taught by means of proper education. If willingness to learn is a quality, it also implies that discipline is at the heart of the matter. Of course, in some cases instilling this quality in children can be relatively easy, while in other cases it might be a much more difficult task.

If one studies the emotional aspects of concentration, one finds that the stratified nature of learning also applies here. The first step is that a child must be taught to listen to and obey ordinary commands. Unless a child has learned to obey his parents in his everyday life, there is no way that he can be taught to follow commands in a more formal learning situation—the second step. He will not listen to his parents, and even less to his teacher, when instructed to sit still, stop fidgeting, stop annoying other children, and remain seated.

The third step, after a child has been taught to remain seated and sit still, is that he must be taught to have the correct predisposition toward work. A favorable predisposition toward work consists of the following qualities:

- Motivation and perseverance: A child must be taught to keep on trying even if he does not succeed the first time;

- A positive attitude: A child must be taught to be positive toward his work. He must, in other words, be task orientated and attach value to the end product;

- A sense of responsibility: A child must be taught that there are some things in life that one *has* to do, even though one may not like doing them.

These qualities, motivation, perseverance, a positive attitude, and a sense of responsibility, are all qualities that a person *must* acquire before he becomes suitable to enter the labor market. An adult who does not possess these qualities is bound to be unsuccessful in the labor market. The above three steps which make a child receptive to learning on an emotional level are therefore not only important for the present situation, but also for the future of the child when he eventually leaves school.

As the primary educators of children, a child's parents are responsible for the accomplishment of this most important educational procedure. No teacher or any other person can teach a child to be emotionally receptive to learning—to be willing or even eager to learn. The teacher is responsible—or is supposed to be responsible—for the formal aspects of education, namely subject instruction.

Apart from making the child emotionally receptive toward learning, it is also the duty of parents to make the child *intellectually* receptive for learning. Parents have to ensure that their child is suitably equipped so that he may profit from the subject instruction

offered to him at school. Although there can be no doubt that the
unwise educational practices implemented in schools—such as replacing drilling and repetition with entertainment—have contributed greatly to the deterioration of education as a whole, the role
that parents play in their children's academic achievement may not
be underestimated. The important role of the parents in a child's
school achievement is confirmed by the famous Coleman report in
the U.S., which stated that achievement differences in schoolchildren were accounted for mostly by what the children *brought with
them to school*.[1] Unfortunately, due to the interruption of the child-
rearing traditions, few parents know that they have such a responsibility. And those who have a vague inkling of it, do not know how
to go about accomplishing this task.

The Interruption of Intellectual Traditions

A problem that has become increasingly prevalent among children in recent times, is that they cannot distinguish between left
and right, and also that they find it difficult to cross the middle line.
The consequence is that they have reading, spelling, and writing
problems when they go to school. Although there are many other
telltale signs of a reading problem, a common result of a confusion
between left and right or a difficulty in crossing the middle line is
that children make reversals when they read or write. They often
confuse letters like b and d, either when reading or when writing,
or they sometimes read (or write) words like "rat" for "tar" or "won"
for "now."

The presently most widely accepted explanation for the above-
mentioned problems is that these children suffer from a "neurological dysfunction." Any person who clings to such an explanation
definitely overlooks the golden thread that runs throughout this
book, namely that there is nothing that any human being knows, or
can do, that he has not learned. Of course, he also overlooks the
stratified nature of learning.

The human body consists of two halves, a left side and a right
side. The human brain also has two halves, which are connected by
the corpus callosum. Mindful of the wise words of Immanuel Kant
that man does not see things as they are but as *he* is, it is inevitable
that a person will interpret everything in terms of his own sidedness.
A child or adult who has not learned to interpret correctly in terms
of his sidedness yet, who has not learned to distinguish properly
between left and right, will inevitably experience problems when he

finds himself in a situation where he is expected to interpret sidedness. (See the *Act of Reading* diagram in this chapter—sidedness is one of the "position in space" interpretations.) One such situation, where sidedness plays a particularly important role, is when a person is expected to distinguish between a *b* and a *d*. It is clear that the only difference between the two letters is the position of the straight line—it is either left or right.

It is important to note that people who are confused about left and right cannot use mnemonics or memory aids while reading, as is often advised by experts. Susan Hampshire, for example, advises that children should remember that "left" is the side on which they wear their watch.[2] This never works to improve reading ability. It can be compared to learning a language. One cannot speak a foreign language if one only has a dictionary in that language. One has to *learn* to speak it. In the same way one has to *learn* to interpret sidedness. As all the other skills foundational to reading, the ability to distinguish between left and right must be drummed in so securely that the person can apply it during reading without having to think of it at all.

One of the reasons why reading problems became more and more acute in the foregoing decades, can, just as the increase in behavior problems, be found in the interruption of the child-rearing traditions. One of the things that parents drummed into their children in the past was the ability to distinguish left from right. The interruption of intellectual traditions such as these can be attributed to the idea that the development of the child is mainly a process of maturation, with learning playing no more than a minor supporting role. At birth, it is assumed, everything the child needs to know or be able to do is already in him—it is only slumbering in the child. One only has to wait, because at the right time, everything will happen and a child will know what he has to know and be able to do what he should be able to do. This "process of maturation" is thus viewed as a *natural process,* and therefore it is believed that the process of maturation cannot be *appreciably* speeded up. Any efforts to speed up this process are seen as a waste of time (see also chapter four). In fact, in the past it was even proclaimed that trying to speed up the maturation process could be harmful, as it could lead to learning failure.

The idea that efforts to accelerate the maturation process can be harmful was in all probability derived from empirical research provided by Carleton Washburne and M. V. Morphett. These two seemed to prove that it was a waste of time—and probably harmful, too—to try and teach children with a mental age lower than six and a half, or at least six years, to read. This was in 1929, and the investigation on which their very dubious findings were based was carried out in schools in Winnetka. Afterward, these findings were quoted with amazing regularity for many decades to warn against the dangers of beginning too early with the teaching of reading.[3]

Morphett and Washburne's conclusions were nothing but mere myth—one of many falsehoods over the past few decades that was shouted from the rooftops to unsuspecting parents. Japanese parents in the 1980s provided ample proof of this. According to Sheridan, by the time Japanese children entered first grade, only 1 percent of them could not recognize any Hiragana symbols (Hiragana is one of the Japanese syllabaries). It was not unusual for 4-year-olds to read books entirely in Hiragana.[4] If there were any truth in Morphett and Washburne's conclusions, it would have been difficult to explain why reading problems were nonexistent in Japan, while parents used to teach their children to read at such a tender age. In fact, in the 1980s, "excessive reading," as opposed to a lack of interest in reading, was a far more widely recognized problem in Japan.[5]

Schmidt also points out that an analysis of Morphett and Washburne's original papers reveals—even to a person with no knowledge of statistical procedures—that their inference was based on very scanty evidence indeed and that their generalization was based on very insecure foundations. Nevertheless, the inference of Morphett and Washburne became an established and accepted dogma.[6] In fact, for fear that they might teach their children incorrectly, this dogma later extended to the idea that parents shouldn't teach their preschool children anything.

The preschool phase is the most important learning time in a person's whole life. Parents who do not teach their children anything during these years are not doing them a favor but a gross injustice. Although a recurrence of this wisdom reemerged in the recent past, as a result of the break that occurred in the traditions, modern-day parents have no idea of how to take care of the intellectual needs of their children during this very important time. Today's parents often think that the key that will unlock their children's intellectual abilities lies in the *quantity* of books and educational toys. It is, however, not the quantity that counts, but the *quality*.

A few decades ago there was not the abundance of story books that there are today. Parents were compelled—it was also part of the child-rearing traditions—to tell over and over to their children the few stories which they knew or to read over and over to their children the few books in their possession. They also spent a lot of time teaching their children rhymes and songs. As Susan discovered through her elder son, this over-and-over repetition of the *same* stories and rhymes was not only effective in that it created a "pyramid of repetition," it was also extremely beneficial for the acquisition of *language*.

Soon after Gustav was born, she bought him a book with the story of *Pinocchio*. The book was aimed at 4-year-olds. Except for talking to him continually, she started to read to him from this book when he was only 2- or 3-months-old—as often as she could, over and over and over. She found this very boring, of course. Gustav, however, loved it, and the results of this experiment made all her efforts worthwhile. Not only did he start talking much sooner than most children do, but when he was just over two years, he could recite nearly all the pages from *Pinocchio*. When turning to a new page, one only had to read the first few words on that page and he would recite the rest of the page like a parrot. In itself, this might seem quite useless, but of great importance was that the vocabulary in this book soon became part of his everyday speech. In terms of language development, he was soon miles ahead of his age group. In fact, to this day, his vocabulary and his ability to speak with clarity are quite astounding.

Language also plays a vital role in reading. Its role in reading can be compared to the role of running in the game of soccer. One cannot play soccer if one cannot run. One cannot read a book in a language unless one knows that particular language. Unless one can speak French, one would not be able read French. Similarly, if a child's knowledge of English is poor, then his reading will also be poor. This means that the cause of a reading problem can go even deeper than merely that the foundational skills of reading have not been adequately mastered. If a child's grasp of the English language is inadequate, the only way through which his reading could be improved would be by not only teaching the skills foundational to reading, but by also improving his command of English. Without effectively working at improving his English, the reading ability of the child will *not* improve.

Parents of previous generations spent a lot of time teaching their babies to talk. In that way, they acquired a good command of whatever language the parents spoke. That the loss of this tradition has contributed generously to the explosion in reading problems over the past few decades is certain. According to Hornsby, about 60 percent of dyslexics are late talkers.[7] This clearly indicates that there is a much closer link between a reading problem and the acquisition of language than is generally realized.

Another tradition, which we learned about too late for Susan's elder son to benefit from, but not Jean, the younger, is more physical in nature. Nevertheless, its effect is also intellectual to some extent.

One often hears today of children who have so-called low muscle tone, as well as problems with gross and fine motor coordination. Gross motor coordination is the ability of the child to coordinate his large muscle movements and perform various tasks. As a result, children learn to walk, run, jump, ride a tricycle or a bicycle, balance themselves properly on one or two legs, and to hop on one or two legs. Fine motor coordination is the development of fine muscle coordination for more exacting tasks such as placing blocks one on top of another, doing up buttons or learning to tie shoelaces and, eventually, acquiring an appropriate handwriting.[8] The result of poor development of a child's gross or fine motor coordination is clumsiness, either when performing tasks that require gross or fine motor skills.

When Gustav was still a baby, Susan and her husband followed the same unwise practice that many parents follow today. They often put him in a walking ring. He was very weak and small, and today we are convinced that this practice has contributed to his weakness. Perhaps this was the cause of his clumsy gait. We don't know. If it was, at least they have taken steps to correct it. But they certainly did not repeat this foolish practice with Jean. They followed an old tradition instead. Even before he was two months old, they often placed him on the floor on his stomach and left him in this position for quite some time. The result of this seemingly insignificant procedure is telling. Although Jean is even shorter and not much bigger than Gustav was at the age of four, his body, and especially his back, arms, and hands, are extraordinarily strong. The effort of trying to push himself up as a baby while lying on his stomach, we guess, must have strengthened many muscles that one needs in daily life. Jean, without doubt, will be the last to have problems with gross or fine motor coordination, and definitely not low muscle tone.

Although we thoroughly enjoy and make use of the benefits of our modern world, when it comes to the education of children, we have learned to respect and trust the old child-rearing traditions. Before throwing any of them overboard, one should first try to establish the rationale behind them. One would usually find that there is some very important logic underlying each of them and that children benefit greatly from their faithful application. Our disregard for these traditions in favor of the modern ideas of psychology and psychiatry have, without doubt, caused millions of children to suffer—not only on an emotional level, but also on an intellectual level. In this respect we must perhaps pay attention to the words of Blatt: "We must take all history seriously—the history of what we did right and the history of what we did wrong. People learn from both their successes and their failures.[9]

Notes

1. Kerlinger, F. N., *Foundations of Behavioral Research* (New York: CBS Publishing Ltd., 1986).

2. Hampshire, S., *Every Letter Counts. Winning in Life Despite Dyslexia* (London: Corgi Books, 1991).

3. Schmidt, W. H. O., *Child Development: The Human, Cultural, and Educational Context* (New York: Harper & Row, 1973), 8.

4. Sheridan, E. M., "Reading disabilities: Can we blame the written language?" *Journal of Learning Disabilities,* vol. 16(2), 1983, 81-86.

5. Ibid.

6. Schmidt, *Child Development,* 8-9.

7. Hornsby, B., *Overcoming Dyslexia* (Johannesburg: Juta and Company Ltd., 1984), 32.

8. Serfontein, G., *The Hidden Handicap* (Sydney: Simon & Schuster, 1990), 43.

9. Blatt, B., "Bandwagons also go to funerals," *Journal of Learning Disabilities,* vol. 12(4), 1979, 222-224.

16.

The Road That Conquers Death

"What is the meaning of man's existence?"

The question, "What is man?" is actually a question of seeking to know oneself, because the alternative is "Who am I?" Similarly, the question seeking the meaning of man's existence is a far more personal question than it might seem at first sight. The alternative form of the question "What is the meaning of man's existence?" is *"Why am I here?"* Every person is at some time of his or her life somehow confronted by this daunting question.

For psychologist Abraham Maslow, meaning is experienced by the self-actualized, growth-motivated person who delights in using his creative powers for their own sake, and who can affirm himself and simultaneously transcend himself through so-called "peak experiences." For Viktor Frankl, meaning is experienced by responding to the demands of the situation at hand, discovering and committing oneself to one's own unique task in life, and by allowing oneself to experience or trust in an ultimate meaning—which one may or may not call God. For Abraham Heschel, man experiences his life as meaningful when he lives in God's presence—not simply by encountering God in the world, but primarily by serving God in everyday life, infusing every moment with the spirit of God, and by dedicating himself to ends outside himself. For Paul Tillich, man can choose to make his life meaningful by surrendering in faith and love to Jesus. By opening to Jesus and experiencing His acceptance and forgiveness, one experiences the joy and freedom of new being and the courage to be oneself.[1]

To a large extent, the answer any person will give to this *why* question will be determined by his view on *what* man is. For example, the evolutionist view of man is that man is a stimulus-response mechanism. It is believed that man's behavior is an automatic reaction to stimuli from his environment or to his inner urges and impulses—in the same way that the animal's behavior is regulated by his instincts. Like the animal, man has no control over his behavior. When such a view of man is accepted, it is naturally regarded as meaningless, even *senseless*, to ponder the meaning of man's existence. Freud, therefore, wrote in a letter to Princess Bonaparte, "The moment a man questions the meaning and value of life he is sick."[2]

The other extreme of the evolutionist view is the existentialist view of man, which overemphasizes the freedom of man. Jean Paul Sartre, one of the foremost existentialist philosophers, said that man is *doomed* to freedom. As soon as one accepts the idea of absolute freedom, it implies that absolute truth cannot and does not exist. If I believe that only *A* is true, it deprives me of the freedom to believe that *B* is true. Similarly, because they restrict man's freedom, all values and norms, principles, and objectives are also denied. According to the existentialist view, human existence is temporary with death as the final end. Therefore man must live for the moment—for the here and now. This implies that man's meaning is rooted in the here and now.

If the meaning of man's existence consists of living only for the moment, his life becomes meaningless and therefore also senseless. As an example of such a senseless life one can refer to the hippies, who rejected the Establishment in the late 1960s and turned, among others, to Zen Buddhism. But their version of Zen Buddhism was a far cry from the discipline of the Japanese Zen monks. Buddhist beliefs and customs were twisted to justify trips into emotion, sensuality, sensation, and self-indulgent abuse of drugs, liquor, and sex.[3]

If one should apply any of these two diverse views of man to our topic of discussion—the child with ADHD—it would, in both cases, imply that parents have to accept their children's behavior, and should not try to change it. According to adherents of the evolutionist view of man the child is a stimulus-response mechanism who cannot be held responsible for his actions. Adherents to the existentialist view, on the other hand, see no reason for any change. The child must be granted complete freedom to do as he pleases. Of course, both views ignore the wisdom of Goethe, that if we take a person as he is, we make him worse; if we take him as he ought to be, we help him become it.

The question *What is the meaning of man's existence?* is, like the question *What is man?*, not an easy question to answer. There is probably also no single answer. To study this riddle—which probably confronts every person at some time in his life—it would perhaps again be appropriate to reword the well-known question of Immanuel Kant. One could start the discussion with the question, *What does man need to live a meaningful life?*

Man's Search for Meaning

From a practical point of view, man's physical needs are his most important needs, but from a perspective of experience, man's need for *meaning* in his life is probably the most pressing. The question is, however, in what *way* can this need be satisfied?

The late Dr. Victor Frankl, who earned fame for his books concerning the meaning of life, demonstrated that meaning cannot coincide with being (the here and now); meaning must be *ahead* of being. He learned this truth while he was a prisoner of war in Germany during World War II. "Meaning sets the pace for being," he wrote. "Existence falters unless it is lived in terms of transcendence towards something beyond itself."[4] This implies that life can only be meaningful if one has a *purpose* to strive for. If one has a purpose, it sets the pace for the here and now. Because one has a purpose in life, it forces one to *do* something every day in order to achieve this objective. A traveler who knows where he is heading, can walk forward purposefully and in this way he can—step by step—come closer to his destination. The fact that he has a goal to aim for gives meaning to his journey. A person who does not have a future purpose can be compared to a traveler who does not know where he is going.

Life offers a legion of purposes that one can strive for. A child's purpose can be to complete school. Thereafter his purpose can be to get a degree or a diploma which enables him to go to university or college. One person's purpose can be to become wealthy. Another can perhaps aim at setting up a charity organization. Another person, on the other hand, can have as his aim to be a famous artist, or a musician. When two people get married, their mutual purpose can be to make each other happy. When blessed with children, it can be their purpose to give their children a decent education. Whatever a person's purpose in life is, he can only accomplish it if he, like the traveler, exerts himself to get closer—step by step—to his destination.

As soon as a person has set a purpose for himself, a continual appeal is directed at him to achieve this objective. If he responds to this appeal by actively working to reach this goal, it implies that he takes *responsibility* for his own life. Every person is responsible for the fulfillment of the specific meaning of his own life. However, because we always share our lives with those of others, no human being can experience meaning without the help and support of others. A child cannot complete school without the assistance of his parents and teachers, the businessman cannot achieve his objectives without clients, an artist cannot become famous without people who admire his artwork, and one cannot make one's spouse happy if he or she is disinterested in you. This implies that each person is not only responsible for himself, but also for *others*. And because a child needs to be *taught* to accept responsibility for his own life—as well as that of others—parents are especially responsible for their children.

It is only by setting goals in the future that one's earthly life can have meaning. The problem with these goals or objectives that one sets in the future, however, is the fact that there is no certainty about the future. No human being knows what tomorrow or the day after tomorrow will bring. Nobody knows whether he will be alive when the sun rises the next morning. Indeed, the fact that there *is* the finality of death, bringing one's life to an inescapable end, without the slightest idea *when* this final end will come, is precisely what brings uncertainty into one's life.

Throughout human history, people have refused to accept the finality of death. Death brings an unacceptable, sudden interruption to one's work, plans, and relationships. Though the inscription on many tombstones reads "Rest in Peace," the truth of the matter is that most people do not welcome the peaceful rest of the grave. They would rather be alive and productive. It is therefore not surprising that the subject of death and afterlife has always been a matter of intense concern and speculation. After all, the death rate is still one per person. Each of us, at the appointed time, will face the grim reality of death.[5]

To conquer death is man's greatest hope, and therefore also his final and overarching purpose. Most of us want to live as long as possible. There are, however, very few who succeed in living very long. The Bible mentions quite a number of people who became extraordinarily old. Even in our times it sometimes happens that a person succeeds in evading death for an astoundingly long time. One of the most astonishing examples of this is the Chinese Lee Cheng-yuen, who reportedly died in 1930 at the age of 252.[6] Emperor Shih Wan Ti looked desperately for a magic potion for longevity, while the Egyptian monarchs built their pyramids and placed household utensils in graves because of a wistful hope that death is not the final end of all life. This hope is not only an historical phenomenon, but also the hope of modern man. There are, for example, those who consider a recipe for immortality as the most important goal of the humanistic ideal, the so-called "New World":

> Once we get off the finite surface of the planet earth and are capable of living in potentially infinite orbital space, there is no reason to have a finite life-span. As engineers of our own body chemistry we can disable the genes that dictate the termination of our life-span, as scientists have already demonstrated with plants and animals. There is no inherent limit to the "Lebensraum" (living space) in orbital space as there is on our planetary surface.

> The life-span of each organism is determined by the environment to which it has adapted. The new environment will be our imagination, which we can only fill if we live forever. We have to be immortal. There is no inherent limit to our imagination as long as there is time and space. The incentive to be a member in good standing in society is the pursuit of immortality. Humankind's social activity, ultimately its urge to mate, is an instinct, just like the instinct to live. If the purpose of society is to protect and enhance the well-being of its members, then providing the means to achieve immortality should be one of its highest priorities. The "New World" must provide individuals with access to the experts, the education and the means to achieve immortality. The difference between our present world based on the formation and protection of family, tribe, nation and the "New World" is that the latter must have as its goal the pursuit of individual immortality.[7]

Throughout the centuries, the most common method whereby man has tried to achieve this final purpose—to conquer death—has been through professing a religion. The Christian religion is unique in that it is believed that death had already been conquered through the death and resurrection of Christ.

By committing himself to a religion, a person places his hope on a supernatural being or power, to whom he hopes to return after his earthly death. The ancient Greeks, for example, believed that the souls of the dead go to the underworld where their god Pluto was believed to reign. This commitment to a religion forces man to accept an authority *higher* than himself.

The religions best known to Westerners are Christianity and Judaism. Islam, however, is also much closer to Christianity and Judaism than is generally realized. All three religions confess the same God—the God of Abraham. Christianity and Judaism, however, go their separate ways when Christians confess that Jesus was the long-awaited Messiah, while Jews continue to await the coming of the Messiah or at least a messianic age. Muslims, on the other hand, believe that Mohammed and Jesus were both messengers of God. Jesus, according to them, was a messenger to his fellow Jews.

Man's hope or faith that he can achieve this final purpose, namely that he can conquer death—or that it has already been conquered—makes it possible for him to, just like the traveler, purposefully undertake the road to his final destination. His *final purpose,* his hope for or faith in an afterlife, gives final meaning to his earthly existence. This final purpose to which a person strives, exhorts him—just like the smaller objectives and goals in his life—to be *responsible,* not only to himself, but also to his spouse, children, employer, society, and also to God, or to whatever authority he might believe in.

When Man's Spiritual Need Is Denied

The deliberation in the previous section, as well as in the one to follow, should *not* be seen as an attempt to convince or prove that all roads lead to Rome, but merely as an attempt to demonstrate that man indeed has a *spiritual need*—the need to conquer death. It is also an attempt to demonstrate that this need can only truly be satisfied through *religion*—defined here as (1) the worship of God or a *higher* authority than man himself, which (2) creates the expectation of the possibility of an *afterlife* and (3) inevitably urges one to be accountable and responsible.

As stated in chapter eleven, the existence of emotional, intellectual, and spiritual needs cannot be directly demonstrated, but their existence can be demonstrated *indirectly* by studying the effect or effects on people if they were to be neglected or ignored. As we have seen in chapters eleven and twelve, insufficient discipline results in insecurity and behavior problems. In chapter thirteen we have discovered that a child, who is insufficiently loved, deteriorates emotionally and even physically. If he is rejected, receiving no love at all, it can even result in death. In chapters fourteen and fifteen we explored the results of insufficient or ineffective learning, i.e., of neglected intellectual needs. This can lead to "learning disabilities" such as dyslexia, which can eventually destroy a person's feelings of self-worth and lead to unemployment. The question that now calls for an answer is, *What happens when the need for an eternal life through religion is neglected?*

It is the desire to *live* that prompts a person to embrace a religion. It is not surprising, therefore, that the most notable consequence of a neglect of religion is the desire to die. A decrease in the practice of religion should therefore lead to an increase in suicide. That this is indeed so has been demonstrated through research and through experience in real life.

Prior to the 1970s, the province of Quebec had a relatively low suicide rate. In the mid-1970s it ranked fourth among the Canadian provinces with a rate well below the Canadian average.[8] In recent years, however, Quebec's suicide rate stands well above the national average. At present, suicide is the leading cause of death for men aged fifteen to twenty-nine in Quebec.[9]

In their study, Krull and Trovato argued that this phenomenon is an outcome of the rapid modernization of Quebec since the late 1950s. Since the late 1950s the society has been transformed from a rural, deeply religious society with a large closely-knit family system to an urban-industrial society that has rapidly abandoned the Church and other traditional forms of regulation in people's lives. In the course of significant social and economic transformation, individualism—the tendency for the individual to rely more on the self for personal meaning and conduct in life—has gradually replaced tradition as the dominant orientation in people's lives. The individual has become increasingly independent, detached from, and less subordinate to traditional forms of integration and social control, such as the church, the extended family, and the parish. As a result of this tendency, the individual is in a general state of isolation from the collectivity, thereby making the individual more prone to despair in times of personal crises, with an increased likelihood of suicide.[10]

George Comstock and Kay Partridge from Johns Hopkins University School of Public Health found that those who did not attend church were four times more likely to commit suicide than those who frequently attended church. Steve Stack, Professor at Wayne State University, also found that non-church attendants were four times more likely to kill themselves than were regular attendants, and that church attendance predicted suicide rates more effectively than *any* other factor, including unemployment. According to Stack suicide seems to be a less acceptable alternative for the religiously committed because of their belief in a moral accountability to God. In addition, the foundational religious belief in an afterlife, eternal justice, and the possibility of condemnation reduces the appeal of self-destructive behavior.[11]

In an attempt to confirm the above studies, we compared the general religiousness of countries with their suicide rates. Countries with exceptionally low suicide rates are Kuwait (0.3 per 100,000 each year), Mexico (± 2 per 100,000), Ecuador (± 4) and Israel (6). These countries are quite dissimilar, except for their *religious commitment*. Kuwait is a Muslim country; Islam is a religion that strictly forbids suicide. In Mexico, as well as in Ecuador, the Catholic Church is still a powerful force, whereas Israel consists of Jews, Muslims, and Christians. Countries with exceptionally high suicide rates, on the other hand, are all countries where the Church and religious traditions have at one time or other been pushed into the background, sometimes forcefully by a Communist Regime. Countries with suicide rates of twenty or more per 100,000 per year include Hungary, Denmark, East Germany, Austria, Finland, Switzerland, West Germany, and Czechoslovakia. Hungary's suicide rate at present is 38.6 per 100,000 and Finland's 27.3.

As noted in previous chapters, Communism was not the only force responsible for the destruction of religion. Psychology and psychiatry have worked equally hard toward the same goal, not only by attacking schools (words used by psychiatrist Ralph Truitt), but also religious institutions:

> The assault on religion continued, this time with direct hits on its institutions. In 1967, psychologist William Coulson, working under the auspices of Carl Rogers, introduced humanistic psychology and "nondirective counseling" to some two dozen religious orders. The results of his "research" was the complete destruction of the religious order of the Sisters of the Immaculate Heart of Mary and their 59 schools in less than a year and a half.

> In 1993, Coulson, realizing the evil he had caused, recanted his psychiatric philosophy and confessed his sins in a statement to the press:

> "We corrupted a whole raft of religious orders on the West Coast in the '60s by getting nuns and priests to talk about

their distress. . . . The IHMs (Sisters of the Immaculate Heart of Mary) had some 60 schools when we started; at the end, they had one. There were some 560 nuns when we began. Within a year after our first interventions, 300 of them were petitioning Rome to get out of their vows. They did not want to be under anybody's authority, except the authority of their empirical inner selves.

"We did similar programs for the Jesuits, for the Franciscans, for the Sisters of Providence of Charity, and for the Mercy Sisters. We did dozens of Catholic religious organizations.

"We provoked an epidemic of sexual misconduct among clergy and therapists. . . .

"The net outcome of sex education, styled as Rogerian encountering, is more sexual experience.

"Humanistic psychotherapy, the kind that has virtually taken over the Church of America . . . dominates so many forms of aberrant education like sex education, and drug education. . . ."[12]

We also examined the incidence of suicide among Buddhists. Buddhism is not a religion in the pure sense of the word, as it does not worship any god. Its proponents refer to it as a "philosophy of awakening." The way through which Buddhists believe they can conquer death is by means of *reincarnation*. This philosophy does not exempt one from responsibility as it is *also* believed that the individual will reap in a next life what he sows in this life. Suicide is rejected because it interrupts the natural cycle of new lives and therefore postpones *nirvana* (a dimension transcending time and space).

We were therefore surprised to find that suicide in the Buddhist-majority of Sri Lanka is extremely high. At the time of writing, Sri Lanka was still home to one of the world's longest and most vicious civil wars, where terrorist bombs, the shelling of civilians, and thousands of nighttime murders have left 50,000 people dead over the last decade. But terrorists were not the only concern. In a study in 1996, it was found that forty-six suicides per 100,000 of the population were committed each year, making it the highest suicide rate in the world.[13] One village of just four hundred souls in northwest Sri Lanka recorded twenty-five suicides in 1997. Two-thirds of the dead were under thirty years of age.[14]

Some attribute the cause of Sri Lanka's high suicide rate to the belief in reincarnation that makes suicide appear less final. An important idea of Buddhism is to recognize the cause of suffering and to put an end to suffering for oneself and for others as well. However, when faced by heavy suffering, the prospect of another life can seem like an attractive option. This view seems to be confirmed by the situation in Tibet. Since 1949, when Chinese troops invaded Tibet, until 1979, 1.2 million Tibetans have died as a result of the Chinese invasion. Of this figure, little over nine thousand (seventy-five of every one hundred thousand who died) died by their own hands. On the other hand, even in the darkest moments of the Jews' existence—the Holocaust—suicide was rare and, among halachic Jews, virtually non-existent.[15] The belief in a *one* and *only* life held by Judaism, Christianity and Islam, as well as the belief that this one and only life determines one's participation in an afterlife, seems to play a big role in making suffering more tolerable. Of course, even in a one and only life suffering can be tolerable only if it has *meaning*. As Frankl said, man is ready and willing to shoulder any suffering as soon and as long as he can see meaning in it.[16] The Scriptures provide ample meaning to suffering. In 2 Corinthians 12:10, for example, it is stated, "That is why, for Christ's sake, I delight in weaknesses, in insults, in hardships, in persecutions, in difficulties. For when I am weak, then I am strong."

Religious commitment does not only reduce suicide, but it also makes for better marriages, better health (even when controlled for smoking) and faster recovery after surgery. In one study, researchers at the Dartmouth College Medical Center studied 232 patients fifty-five years of age or older who were undergoing elective heart surgery in order to determine what particular variables might contribute to survival. The findings led the researchers to conclude that "those without any strength or comfort from religion had almost three times the risk of death as those with at least some strength and comfort." Furthermore, the more religious the patient, the more protected they seemed to be from death after surgery. Of the thirty-seven patients who described themselves as deeply religious, none died. Only 5 percent of those who attended church at least every few months died in the six months following the operation, compared with 12 percent of those who rarely or never did so.[17]

In other studies, religion was found to curtail drug and alcohol abuse. In a national survey of twelve thousand adolescents it was found that the measure of the "importance of religion" to the person was the best predictor in indicating a lack of substance abuse—a result of deeply internalized norms and values.[18]

Research has also consistently shown that religious individuals live longer than the less religious do. Solomon said in Proverbs 9:10-11: "The fear of the Lord is the beginning of wisdom, and knowledge of the Holy one is understanding. For through me your days will be many, and years will be added to your life." A study by Diana Zuckerman and Stan Kasl of Yale University—as well as many other studies—indicated that this promise in Proverbs is not an idle one. In their study over a two year period of a population living outside New Haven, Connecticut, factors such as age, marital status, education, income, race, gender, the subject's health, and previous hospitalizations were all controlled for. In addition, the researchers assessed each subject's frequency of attendance at religious services, reports of how personally religious they were, and importance of religion as a source of strength. After the two year follow-up period, the less religious were found to have mortality levels twice those of the more religious.[19]

Noteworthy research also demonstrated that psychiatrists who are more likely to be atheists commit suicide *five times* the rate of the population at large, and are overrepresented in studies concerning alcoholic abuse and drug abuse among physicians. Marriage is another sore spot. One study found that they had the shortest marriages, were most likely to "carry on and scream" during family quarrels, and were most likely to have problems due to extramarital affairs.[20]

When one has little time, one is often inclined to neglect the religious education of one's children. We hope that the above-mentioned studies and real-life events will encourage parents to take this aspect of their children's education very seriously.

Notes

1. Marks, T., *The Meaning of Life according to Seven Philosophers, Psychologists and Theologians* (Tufts University: An independent study project, 1972).

2. Freud, E. L. (ed.), *Letters of Freud* (New York: Basic Books Inc., 1960), cited in V. E. Frankl, *Psychotherapy and Existentialism* (Harmondsworth, Middlesex: Penguin Books, 1973), 30.

3. Raschke, C. A., *The Interruption of Eternity: Modern Gnosticism and the Origins of the New Religious Consciousness* (Chicago: Nelson-Hall,

1980), cited in I. H. Horn, *The Implications of the New Age Thought for the Quest of Truth: A Historical Perspective* (University of South Africa: Unpublished DEd-Thesis, 1996), 49.

4. Frankl, V. E., *Psychotherapy and Existentialism*, 22-23.

5. Bacchiocchi, S., *Immortality or Resurrection? A Biblical Study on Human Nature and Destiny*, Chapter IV.

6. Reid, D., *Guarding the Three Treasures* (London: Simon & Schuster, 1993).

7. Schickentanz, A., alfred@well.com, website.

8. Krull, C., & Trovato, F., "The quiet revolution and the sex differential in Quebec's suicide rates: 1931-1986," *Social Forces*, vol. 72, 1994, 1121-1147.

9. "Quebec has top suicide rate: Government vows to fight problem," *Medical Post*, vol. 34, 24 February 1988, 36.

10. Krull & Trovato, "The quiet revolution and the sex differential in Quebec's suicide rates."

11. Larson, D., Milano M. G, & Barry, C., "Religion: The forgotten factor in health care." *The World & I*, vol. 11, 1996: 292.

12. Coulson, W., "How I wrecked the I.H.M. nuns," *The Latin Mass*, Special edition, 12-16, cited in T. Röder, V. Kubillus & A. Burwell, *Psychiatrists: The Men Behind Hitler* (Los Angeles: Freedom Publishing, 1994), 317-318.

13. McGirk, J., "Suicide soars in the midst of 'paradise' isle gets a bad name," *Independent on Sunday*, 8 December 1996, 15.

14. Perera, J., "Health—Sri Lanka: Devastatingly high suicide rate needs research," *Inter Press Service English News Wire*, 10 July 1998.

15. Breitowitz, Y., "Does Judaism ever sanction suicide, and may a physician or any third," *Moment*, 31 December 1996.

16. Frankl, *Psychotherapy and Existentialism*, 34.

17. Larson, Milano & Barry, "Religion: The forgotten factor in health care."

18. Ibid.

19. Ibid.

20. Wiseman, B., *Psychiatry: The Ultimate Betrayal* (Los Angeles: Freedom Publishing, 1995), 45-46.

17.

The "Religion" of Modern Man

Rudyard Kipling once wrote, "East is East, and West is West, and never the twain shall meet." But that can no longer be said, now that a pantheistic Eastern philosophy is spreading like wildfire into the Western world. The primary vehicle for this transmission of ideas has been the New Age Movement.[1] Due to its massive influence in the West, this movement simply cannot be omitted in any discussion of religion.

The New Age Movement has many subdivisions, but it is generally a collection of Eastern-influenced metaphysical thought systems, a conglomeration of theologies, hopes, and expectations held together with an eclectic teaching of salvation, of correct thinking, and correct knowledge. It is a theology of feel-goodism, universal tolerance, and moral relativism.[2] The Movement has no official leader, headquarters, nor membership list, but instead is a network of groups working toward specific goals.[3] Publications, which list the numerous cooperating groups, are the *Spiritual Community Guide,* and *The New Age Magazine,* with thousands of listings. New Agers claim that all mind science groups are a part of the *new age.*

They also include various occult groups, mystic religions, witchcraft organizations, pagan religions, ecological organizations, neopolitical and secular organizations. In the U.S. and Canada, over 10,000 organizations are identified as New Age, such as Amnesty International, Greenpeace, The Sierra Club, Zero Population, The Guardian Angels, and thousands of other secular and religious organizations. Before the Jonestown, Guyana massacre in 1978, which left 914 people dead, Rev. Jim Jones' Peoples Temple was also listed as a New Age "Spiritual Center" in the *Spiritual Community Guide.* Other groups synonymous with the New Age are The Age of Aquarius, The Aquarian Conspiracy, The Human Potential Movement, The Holistic Movement, Humanistic Psychology, and a host of others.[4]

The ideas on which the New Age Movement is founded are not new. Many of its themes lead back to Gnosticism, a mystical movement in the early days of the church which claimed that man's spirit is good and can be developed into eternal life. The first book of John was written to rebuke the heresy of Gnosticism.

The New Age spirituality is an eclectic stance that borrows from a large variety of spiritual religions or spiritual traditions, such as Hinduism and Buddhism (a watered-down version of both Hinduism and Buddhism, it must be added). In the words of New Age author, Nevill Drury, the view is, "There can be no final 'revelation,' no single path to the Godhead, for 'God' is everywhere—potentially available to all."[5] Yet, although professing a broad-minded openness to all religions, it rejects Judeo-Christian beliefs as well as their attending moral values.[6]

New Agers believe that "all is one." Everything and everyone is interrelated and interdependent. Ultimately, there is no real difference between humans, animals, rocks, or even God. Since New Agers believe that "all is one," the next logical assumption would be that "all is god." If "all is one" and "all is god," then it must be concluded that "we are gods." We are, according to New Agers, ignorant of our divinity. We are "gods in disguise."[7] In New Age thought, God did not create humankind; humankind creates God. Starhawk, author of *The Spiral Dance: A Rebirth of the Ancient Religion of the Great Goddess*, for example, asserts that the goddess "exists, *and* we create Her."[8]

The New Age Movement is striving for a "New World," in which people would live together in divine harmony. Within this hoped-for harmony there will be economic unity. One of the main goals is to bring to the forefront a one-world leader called "The Christ"[9] who will, according to New Age principles, guide the world into a single harmonious economic whole. It is also hoped that this leader will unite the world into a spiritual unity—that is, a one-world religion.[10]

One of the most celebrated demonstrations of unity and public relations occurred on 16-17 August 1988. Over 80 million New Agers unified themselves for what was called the largest assembly of mass meditation in history. Widely reported by the news media, the "Harmonic Convergence," also referred to as the "Planetary Surrender," occurred simultaneously in nearly every nation and major city.

Led and organized largely by 144,000 shamans, witches, witch doctors and a whole assortment of New Age mystics, they joined in a period of meditation for the release of "spiritual forces" which would bring about their desire for "one world government and world religion."[11]

For the most part, the New Age Movement espouses evolution, both of body and spirit. Man is developing and will soon leap forward into new spiritual horizons. Many New Age practices are designed to push one ahead into that horizon. Some of them are astral projection, which is training your soul to leave your body and travel around and contact spirits so they may speak through you or guide you.[12] Other supernatural sources for spiritual growth and healing include past-life regression, dream therapy, fire-walking, crystal power, and pyramid power.[13] As Chesterton wrote, "When a man ceases to believe in God, he does not believe in nothing, he believes in anything."[14]

There are no absolute truths in New Age thinking. Because the average New Ager believes himself to be divine, he can create his own reality. If, for example, a person believes that reincarnation is true—which has appeal to many New Age thinkers—that's fine because that is his reality. If someone he knows doesn't believe in it, that is all right too because that is someone else's reality. Each person can have a reality for himself that "follows a different path."[15] It must be added, however, that reincarnation in the New Age dictionary differs conspicuously from what is said on this subject by (true) Buddhism and Hinduism. According to these philosophies the individual will reap in a next life what he sows in this life. This idea is clearly not part of New Age thinking. Because New Agers believe themselves to be divine, they can decide for themselves about matters regarding morality, belief, and behavior. Morality thus becomes relative and subjective, as New Age author Shirley MacLaine asserts:

> If a child steals to live, if a man kills to protect his family, if a woman aborts a fetus rather than give birth to an unwanted child, if a terrorist murders because he has been raised all his life to believe that killing is his right and proper duty—who is evil? And if a person kills "simply" out of hatred or greed, *he* perceives his motives as *his need*—others make the judgement that his act is "evil."[16]

MacLaine should perhaps learn from history. As Chandler says, "History provides evidence that relative standards of morality breed chaos and—ultimately—the downfall of society."[17]

Influenced by humanistic psychology, New Age thinkers view self-fulfillment as the "highest responsibility." Seen in the light of moral relativism, however, self-fulfillment can be used to justify parents who put their own interests before their duty to their children. Promiscuous sex can be justified; many other forms of immoral and/or amoral behavior, which are harmful to one's fellow human beings (and to nature), can also be justified.[18]

The New Age Movement Finds Its Way to America

The renewed interest in mysticism did not come from nowhere. The New Age Movement started in 1890 in Europe—about the same time that Wundt's "new" psychology was attracting disciples—and got its name from A. J. Orage's theoretical journal, *New Age*. Orage was a Theosophist, a sect that dates back to about 1875 and adheres to a "religious" stew consisting of aspects of Buddhism and Brahmanism, reincarnation, multiple "lives," fatalism, and pessimism. Neill (see chapter four) and Freud took a great liking to Orage's *New Age* journal, and also wrote articles for the publication. Under the influence of a fanatical anti-Semite, Major General J. F. C. Fuller, and occultist/satanist Aleister Crowley, the Theosophy/New Age movement was taken into the nightmare world of drugs, intoxication, and euphoria, resulting in Crowley's "Ordo Templis Orientalis" drug and "sex magic" group in London.[19]

Another influential figure in New Age thinking was Freud's Swiss countryman, the well-known psychologist Carl Gustav Jung. Jung's psychology is rooted in mysticism, Gnosticism, and occultism.[20] In 1916, safe within the borders of a neutral Switzerland while Europe raged with war, Jung gathered his disciples in Zurich and gave a talk that formalized the founding of his own cult, which he called the Psychological Club. This special group of colleagues and ex-patients heard Jung tell them that the path to personality transformation was through an experience of self-deification (literally experiencing oneself to become Christ or a god) and then overcoming it. The method was his own version of "analysis," with himself or a personally approved colleague—including visionary journeys into the "Land of the Dead" to consult with ancestors. Jung could offer these promises to his disciples because he himself had the experience of becoming a god—or so he reported in a 1925 seminar whose contents were known only to a tight circle within the Jungian analytic community until they were finally published in 1989. In 1913, he said, he had a vision in which he became a combination of Christ and a lion-head deity from an ancient Hellenistic mystery cult.[21]

While simmering in Britain and Switzerland for many decades, New Age thinking received little notice in America until the 1960s, when it finally entered via the "hippie" movement under the guidance of the Frankfurt School in Germany.

The Frankfurt School was founded in 1923 by Georg Lukacs, an avid communist. Like Lenin, his zeal was to eradicate religion and the churches and he harbored a deep hatred of anything Western. In 1919, Lukacs became Deputy Commissar for Culture in the Bolshevik Bella Kun Regime in Hungary. His first order of business in Budapest was to do everything he could to keep people out of churches. He launched an aggressive sex education program, which among other instructed children in "free love," emphasizing the irrelevance of religion, which, he said, deprived people of pleasure. Lukacs' sex education program was modified later by American organizations such as SIECUS and adapted for U.S. schools.[22]

The result of Lukacs' 133-day tenure as Commissar for Culture was quite memorable, as "an immense tidal wave of juvenile delinquents emerged who later were easily conscripted to join terrorist squads, torture prisoners, and help impose a police state."[23] "[The] worldwide overturning of values cannot take place without the annihilation of old values and the creation of new ones by the revolutionaries," Lukacs said.[24]

In 1922, Lukacs left for Germany and took up with a group of radical intellectuals, who founded the Institute for Social Research (ISR), or what became known as the Frankfurt School. The nucleus of the Frankfurt school was a mixture of Marxist ideologists, Freudian sexologists, social and political psychologists, and professional propagandists. Key promoters were Lukacs himself, Antonio Gramsci, Max Horkheimer, Erich Fromm (see chapter ten), Wilhelm Reich, Kurt Lewin, Walter Benjamin, Theodor Adorno, and Herbert Marcuse.[25] Neill was also closely associated with this group.

The larger agenda of the Frankfurt School/ISR was (1) the "abolition of culture," as Lukacs termed it, so as to undermine the Judeo-Christian value structure, and (2) to introduce a "new barbarism"—new cultural icons and ideas that would be sure to divide the population and increase alienation between the younger and older generation. Authoritarian characteristics, such as capitalism, national sovereignty, disciplined children, and rationality were seen as a problem.[26] "The authoritarian family is the authoritarian state in miniature," Reich wrote in 1933. In his book, *The Mass Psychology of Fascism,* he set out specific theses—a list of "to do's." These included:

- The idea that organized religion, particularly Christianity, is a hangover of the authoritarian family ideal which led to Fascism, and that authoritarian moralism must be eradicated.

- A repetition of the Wundtian notion that man was primarily a neurochemical machine and sexual animal.

- The idea that a matriarchy is superior to the paternally orientated family and social structure, and that the feminist agenda must, therefore, be actively pursued.[27]

Many of the Frankfurt School/ISR left for the United States. Fromm and Marcuse went to America in the early 1930s and Horkheimer during World War II.

The Frankfurt School or Institute for Social Research became most influential in America. In 1934, according to historian Martin May, Columbia University's then-president, N.M. Butler, invited the Frankfurt School to affiliate with the University. This affiliation became known as the *International* Institute for Social Research, and a viable affiliation for the Marxists. More than two decades later, for example, Marcuse's *Eros and Civilization* (1955) was published with funding of the Rockefeller Foundation. Beginning with Columbia's Teachers College (the home of Thorndike and Dewey), it was pressed into the hands of student anti-war activists, bringing the Frankfurt School's messianic revolutionary mission to all the American colleges and universities.[28] As we have seen in chapter ten, the ISR, especially Erich Fromm, also gave momentum to the Mental Hygiene Movement.

The main objective of the Marxists was to construct the stereotypical authoritarian composite character as a symbol of intolerance, rigidity, and patriarchal repression to the American public. They used every ploy they could think of, from erotism and feminism to racism, but a key goal was to create an image that compared traditional values unfavorably against the new "revolutionary" *cum* "democratic" man, who supposedly had "vision" and was flexible.[29]

World War II could not have come at a better time. Omitting the fact that *psychiatrists* played a major role in the Holocaust,[30] ISR scholars used World War II crimes to degrade authoritarianism:

Nobody questioned their superiors, claimed Neill, Fromm, Reich, and their cohorts. German and Japanese officials who carried out their leaders' orders had been blind followers of authority, they charged. The chief cause of war became equated with ugly authoritarianism. Gradually the suggestion that children learn to question, and even disobey, their parents, got a foothold in America during the post-War years—first, in professional circles, and then among the public . . .[31]

The anti-authoritarian message made sense. *Do you want your child to grow up to be a Hitler? A Mussolini? A Stalin?* Nobody did. Parents were thus open for new approaches and jumped eagerly at experts such as Spock and Woodward when they came along. But, as Eakman so correctly states, little did they expect the tragedy that would ensue once children became their own masters.[32] Brought up on Spock's permissive ideas, which promoted instant gratification and deviance, the post-War generation was most susceptible to a lifestyle characterized by promiscuity and drug abuse—a lifestyle that was promoted by the Frankfurt School/ISR scholars. They namely opened the door to the New Age occult rituals of satanist Aleister Crowley and psychologist Carl Jung, thereby providing a perfect foundation for the hippie movement.[33]

As time passed, the media—cinema and television—took over from the hippies to propagate the New Age ideas. Public schools have become yet another vehicle. Throughout the West, references to Christianity in handbooks have been replaced by New Age concepts. Prayer is no longer allowed, but New Age practices are. Evolution is a sacred cow, while the story of creation is ridiculed. Should one then be surprised by a 1991 Gallup poll, which indicated that 70 percent of professed Christian students in U.S. public schools no longer attend church two years after graduating?[34]

Parents who want to protect their children from such influences, which in today's world are inescapable, should cultivate spiritual discernment in their children. They should take full responsibility for their children's religious education, assisted, however, by their church. Parents should not shift this essentially parental task onto the school. Assisted by the church, they should provide their children with intellectually solid ammunition which will enable them to defend their beliefs against any contradictory secular or religious beliefs that they may encounter in the schools and in the media.[35] We *have* to teach our children that in traveling to their end-destination they can choose only one of two roads:

> [One] cannot travel both roads at the same time. [One] cannot have one foot on the one road and the other foot on the other road. One leads to life and the other leads to destruction. Nor can [one] travel the broad road and live its lifestyle and receive the benefits of the narrow and straight way.[36]

Summary of Man's Most Important Needs:

1. **Physical Needs:**
   - We must *eat* to satisfy our need for food;
   - We must *drink* to satisfy our need for water;
   - We must *breathe* to satisfy our need for oxygen;
   - We must *sleep* to satisfy our need for rest;
   - We must have *shelter* to satisfy our need for protection.
2. **Emotional Needs:**
   - Our need for security is provided through *discipline*;
   - Our need for acceptance is satisfied through *love*;
   - Our need for dignity is satisfied through *respect*.
3. **Intellectual Need:**
   - The need to know is satisfied by *learning*.
4. **Spiritual Need:**
   - The need to conquer death is (truly) satisfied through *religion*.

Notes

1. Anderson, K., "The New Age Movement," *Probe Ministries*, website.

2. Slick, M., "The New Age Movement," *Christian Apologetics & Research Ministry*, website.

3. "New Age or old occult?" *Biblical Discernment Ministries*, August 1992, website.

4. Robbins, D. A., *Victorious Publications*, 1990, website.

5. Millikan, D., & Drury, N., *Worlds Apart? Christianity and the New Age* (Crows Nest, New South Wales: ABC, 1991), cited in I. H. Horn, *The Implications of the New Age Thought for the Quest of Truth: A Historical Perspective* (University of South Africa: Unpublished DEd-Thesis,

1996), 15.

6. Hunt, cited in "New Age or old occult?", *Biblical Discernment Ministries;* Eakman, B. K., *Cloning of the American Mind: Eradicating Morality through Education* (Lafayette: Huntington House Publishers, 1998), 479.

7. Anderson, "The New Age Movement."

8. Horn, I. H., *The Implications of the New Age Thought for the Quest of Truth.* 215.

9. "New Age or old occult?" *Biblical Discernment Ministries.*

10. Slick, "The New Age Movement."

11. Robbins, *Victorious Publications.*

12. Slick, "The New Age Movement."

13. Horn, *The Implications of the New Age Thought for the Quest of Truth,* 54.

14. Hoyt, K., (ed.), *The New Age Rage* (Old Tappan, NJ: Fleming H. Revell, 1987), cited in Horn, *The Implications of the New Age Thought for the Quest of Truth,* 55.

15. Slick, "The New Age Movement."

16. MacLaine, S., *It's All in the Playing* (Thorndike, Me: Thorndike-Magna, 1987), 222-223.

17. Chandler, R., *Understanding the New Age* (Dallas: Word, 1988), 18.

18. Horn, *The Implications of the New Age Thought for the Quest of Truth,* 103.

19. Eakman, *Cloning of the American Mind,* 227-229, 478.

20. Horn, *The Implications of the New Age Thought for the Quest of Truth,* 109.

21. Noll, R., *New York Times,* 15 October 1994, cited in "Confessions of an analyst," website.

22. Eakman, *Cloning of the American Mind,* 146.

23. Ibid., 147.

24. Ibid.

25. Ibid., 147, 149.

26. Ibid., 149, 155.

27. Ibid., 150-151.

28. Ibid., 153, 155.

29. Ibid., 127.

30. Röder, T., Kubillus, V., & Burwell, A., *Psychiatrists: The Men Behind Hitler* (Los Angeles: Freedom Publishing, 1994); Wiseman, B., *Psychiatry: The Ultimate Betrayal* (Los Angeles: Freedom Publishing, 1995); Eakman, *Cloning of the American Mind,* 169.

31. Eakman, *Cloning of the American Mind,* 168.

32. Ibid., 169.

33. Ibid., 229.

34. *Gallup Report,* 1991, cited in *Focus on the Family.*

35. Wilder-Smith, A. E., *God: To Be or not to Be? A Critical Analysis of Monod's Scientific Materialism* (Stuttgart: Hänssler, 1975), 100, cited in Horn, *The Implications of the New Age Thought for the Quest of Truth,* 213.

36. *New Age Ministries,* website.

18.

Questions and Answers on Discipline

Parents usually have many questions on the topic of discipline. The most pressing ones are answered below. If you have questions other than those dealt with here, or any other questions regarding the topics discussed in this book, you can visit the website at www.audiblox2000.com. The password to get access to the question-answer section is *creators*.

Q *My 6-year-old son will be eligible for school in a few months. He is highly intelligent, but also extremely active and talkative. Does this mean that he will battle to pay attention and concentrate in the classroom?*

A Before answering your question we would like to stress that there is nothing wrong with a child who is active—not even with one who is extremely active. Running, jumping, and climbing are important for a child's motor development. We would have been much more worried if your child had been *hypo*active (the opposite of *hyper*active), as extreme passivity can sometimes be a sign of physical illness. We would then have advised you to take him for a thorough medical checkup, just to make sure that he is not ill. And we would also have advised you to try and raise his activity level by getting him involved in games and activities that require some physical exercise. There is also nothing wrong with a talkative child. It is an indication that his language is probably up to standard.

If your child does not cope in the classroom, his activity level and talkativeness as such are not to blame. A lack of discipline would be a more probable cause.

The difference between a disciplined and an undisciplined child is not that the former is passive and quiet while the latter is active and talkative. The *only* difference is that the former knows that there are boundaries and what they are, while the latter does not.

The former knows that there is a time and a place for being active and talkative, and a time and a place to sit still and/or be quiet. As it is stated in Ecclesiastes 3:1, "There is a time for everything, and a season for every activity under the sun." Verse 3:7 states explicitly that there is "a time to be silent and a time to speak." If this is taught to children from a young age, they will not have a problem sitting still in class and listening to the teacher when it is expected from them.

Our everyday life provides ample situations to teach our children to differentiate between situations where a certain action will be appropriate and situations where the same action will be inappropriate. Unfortunately many parents don't do this anymore. Children are allowed to run and climb wherever and whenever they please. They are also allowed to butt into adults' conversations. And if they happen to do exactly the same in the classroom, then we think that there is something wrong with them—that they suffer from ADHD. It certainly does not make sense.

Traditionally, children were not allowed to butt into an adult conversation. We were raised according to this view. It did not mean that adults never spoke to children. On the contrary. We both grew up in South Africa in a time before televisions were around, and therefore our generations were very dependent on adults to keep us busy. But we knew that when adults were interacting with each other, we had to keep quiet or go and play somewhere else. The result of this was that it *also* taught us not to interrupt a teacher while she was teaching.

If you have taught your child to differentiate between situations in which being active and talkative is acceptable and those in which it is not acceptable, you need not have any sleepless nights about him going to school. If, however, you have neglected to do this, we suggest that you start doing so immediately.

Of course the appropriateness of certain behaviors, such as stealing, does not depend on situations. Stealing is always wrong—full stop.

Q *Many people are of the opinion that the biblical "rod" should be interpreted figuratively and not literally. According to Dr. Ross Campbell, author of "How to Really Love Your Child," the rod was really a shepherd's staff, which was used to firmly, but kindly, guide the sheep.*[1] *Others say that the rod should be interpreted as the Law, not a stick with which to hit children.*

The statistics, such as those quoted in chapters six and twelve, and many others too, clearly indicate that those who interpret the rod figuratively should reconsider their view. The increase in youth violence and numerous other youth problems throughout the world relate directly to the abolition of corporal punishment.

We have been witness to hundreds of children who were cured from ADHD, ODD, CD, and Tourette's syndrome. As soon as loving discipline—which includes the rod of reproof—is brought into homes in the proper way, problems like these disappear. A case study of one such child, who used to have nearly every symptom of all of these four disorders, is discussed in chapter nineteen.

Susan, who at present belongs to a small minority of South African parents who have not fallen for the psychological child-rearing gimmicks, can testify to the effectiveness of the biblical rod. Biblical discipline has changed the worst behavior problems or character traits of her sons into their most positive attributes. Gustav, without doubt, would have had Tourette's syndrome if she and her husband did not intervene. But they did and the negative compulsive tics associated with Tourette's syndrome turned into a very positive character trait. Today he is compulsive about getting something right if he has set his mind on it. He will go on and on, practicing endlessly, until he finally succeeds. One sometimes envies his abundance of self-motivation.

Jean, the younger, on the other hand, was very aggressive and hostile from a young age. His anger and temper outbursts started way before the so-called "terrible-two" phase. Although it is human to get angry at times, a child can and should be taught that there are acceptable and unacceptable ways of expressing it. A temper tantrum is unacceptable, as are behaviors like throwing things around in anger.

Discipline has certainly not made Jean less emotional, but he is now inclined to express kind and positive emotions. In fact, he showers all the members of his family with love and of course wants to be showered with love in return. He is also now able to express anger in an appropriate way. Mostly he will tell one that he is upset about something and why, thereby giving one the opportunity to discuss the matter with him. Once in a while, his old and wrong ways of expressing anger still come to the fore, but these incidences, which are addressed on every occasion, are rare and are occurring ever less often and farther apart.

Another positive effect of biblical discipline which parents soon discover after implementation, is that home becomes a peaceful place. Screaming, shouting, and threatening, which are characteristic of homes where modern child-rearing practices are used, are inclined to destroy peace.

Q *What is the difference between proper punishment and child abuse?*

A Biblical spanking is motivated by the love a parent feels for his child, and has as its purpose to bring correction to a child's heart—to drive folly from it. Though a spanking is not intended to be an enjoyable experience either to the child or to the parent, if properly administered it reaps positive and long-lasting benefits.[2] As it is stated in Hebrews 12:11, "No discipline seems pleasant at the time, but painful. Later on, however, it produces a harvest of righteousness and peace for those who have been trained by it."

Child abuse, on the other hand, is motivated by a parent's anger, frustration, or anxiety, and has as its purpose the venting of such feelings. Even one smack motivated by anger is child abuse, as are verbal insults, which are always motivated by anger or frustration. An abusive parent, without doubt, can cause a child to become violent and aggressive or experience sexual difficulties in adulthood. If you would take the time to study the biographies of a few serial killers, you would find that most of them were either abused as children—physically, sexually, or verbally—or were abused in the sense that they were allowed to do as they pleased. As the examples below indicate, a lack of *loving* discipline in childhood seems to be common to most—if not all—serial killers. Although we do not view this fact as mitigation for murder or rape, it certainly makes one think.

Although Richard Ramirez, the so-called "Night Stalker," was "adored as the baby of the family," he received no loving discipline from his "explosive" and "hot-tempered" father. Neither did his siblings. Two of his three brothers, Ruben and Robert, had behavioral problems in school, got into trouble with the law, sniffed glue, stole cars, burglarized homes, and hung around with the wrong kids. Ruben later became a heroin addict, while Richard became a serial killer. At the end of his trial he was given the death sentence— nineteen times.

John Wayne Gacy, Jr., another serial killer, had very strong relations with his mother and sisters, but his father, John Wayne Gacy, Sr., was an abusive alcoholic who physically abused his wife and verbally assaulted his children.

Although described as a very gentle, decent family man, who just happened to be an incorrigible small-time thief, Albert DeSalvo confessed to being the "Boston Strangler." DeSalvo's father was a violently abusive man who regularly beat his wife and children.[3]

Kenneth Bianchi, one of the "Hillside Stranglers," was seemingly not abused physically, sexually, or verbally, but in a sense that he was allowed to get away with murder. He was a compulsive liar by the time he could talk, suffered from idleness and goldbricking, and was prone to temper tantrums and quick to anger.

Charles Schmid, later known as the "Pied Piper," took many chances and lived dangerously, "without much interference" from his foster parents. He had little regard for learning. He stole some tools from his school's machine shop, after which he was suspended. He could have been readmitted, but he never bothered. By the time he was sixteen, he was living in his own quarters on his parents' property and received an allowance of three hundred dollars a month (a large allowance in the 1950s). His foster parents left him to run on his own with a new car and a motorcycle. He spent much of his time on the speedway, picking up girls, and drinking with buddies, although he tended to be a loner.[4]

Q *Don't you think there is a time and a place for time-out and taking away privileges?*

A If time-out and taking away privileges had been effective, behavioral and emotional problems would not be such an issue today. Tragically, the severity and prevalence of these problems are becoming more alarming because the majority of parents have abandoned God's wisdom in favor of the "wisdom" of psychology and psychiatry.

Although we have never seen it to be effective, we could perhaps tolerate the idea of taking away privileges. But we simply can't stomach the idea of sending a child to his room for time-out. This form of punishment smacks of rejection. What message is a parent conveying when he orders a child to go and sit in his room? It can only be something like, "You are not acceptable. In fact you are so bad that I cannot stand the sight of you right now." When a child feels rejected, he feels unloved. Biblical discipline, on the other hand, does not make a child feel rejected or unloved.

Q *For what reasons should a parent spank his child?*

A Before discussing the reasons *why* a spanking should be given, it is perhaps necessary to mention occasions when a spanking is *not* appropriate. (1) A spanking should never be given to try and force the child to do something that he is not able to do because of *age*.[5] You cannot spank a 6-month-old baby for not lying still while being diapered. (2) One also does not spank a child for something he *cannot do*. If a child truly cannot read, for example, even holding a gun to his head will not make him read. Neither will a spanking. (3) Nor does one spank a child for something he does not know. Unless you have instructed a child properly, you cannot spank him for erring. If he has never received instruction that stealing is wrong, you cannot spank him if he steals. (4) Accidents are also not a reason for a spanking, for example, when a child unintentionally breaks something or unintentionally hurts someone. (5) Lastly, one should *never* spank a child when one's emotions are out of control.

A spanking is appropriate for three reasons only. The first is *willful disobedience* and the second is *wrong attitude*. By teaching a child to obey his parent with a right and cooperating attitude, a parent is preparing his child to eventually obey God with a right attitude: "He has showed you, O man, what is good. And what does the Lord require of you? To act just and to love mercy and to walk humbly with your God" (Micah 6:8).

A child is willfully disobedient when he deliberately disobeys his parents' commands or instructions. It is important to have a clear understanding of the difference between what a child is *unable* to do and what a child *will not do*. If a 2-year-old is asked to answer the telephone and does not, this is not willful disobedience because his age limits the physical ability or comprehension to obey. However, if a normal 2-year-old child is told to "come here" but refuses and goes in an opposite direction, ignoring the parent, that is willful disobedience. It is clear to the parent that the child is able to "come here," but will not.[6]

Obedience should be *prompt, complete,* and *unquestioned*. Children should learn that their parents mean what they say, and parents should expect their children to obey the *first* time they speak. If a parent allows his child to obey him only after he has threatened or scolded, the child is going to wait for the threat or scolding before he obeys. The child will also be unable to obey his teacher—he will wait for a threat or a shout. And don't be surprised if he one day fails to follow the instructions of his employer.

The importance of *complete* obedience is seen in the story of the partial obedience of King Saul. God had commanded him to utterly destroy the Amalekites, including their livestock. When Saul was confronted by Samuel after the battle, he was asked if he had fully obeyed God. As Saul was uttering an affirmative reply, Samuel heard the bleating of sheep in the background. When asked about this, Saul justified his disobedience by saying he had kept them back to offer in sacrifice to God. Samuel answered: "To obey is better than sacrifice, and to heed is better than the fat of rams." The consequence of this partial obedience resulted in the kingdom being taken from him[7] (see 1 Samuel 15). What this means is that, if a parent has given his child a command to do two chores, and he has only done one, he was only partially obedient. Of course, the age of the child should be kept in mind. In the case of a small child, instructions should be simple and only one at a time should be given.

Unquestionable obedience means that the *authority* of the parent may not be questioned. If you have to reason and argue with your child in order to get obedience, you will soon find yourself frustrated and outwitted. However, it does not mean that a child may not ask reasons for a command or an instruction. If he asks for a reason and there is one, give it to him. If there is none and he asks for it, then "because I say so" will be sufficient. There isn't always a logical reason for everything. There isn't a logical reason why the rules of the game of ice hockey are one way and not another. Somebody or some authoritative body decided that the rules should be what they are and if you want to play the game, you have to adhere to these rules. If everybody were allowed to make his own rules, ice hockey would be unplayable. In the same way, the rules of the game of life are not always founded on logic. There are many values and norms, which have been ingrained in Western society for many generations, for which there are no logical reasons. But they make the game of life playable. As more and more children are allowed to make their own rules in the game of life, it is gradually becoming less and less playable. To summarize, a child may ask for reasons for commands and instructions but must accept them without question.

A second good reason for a spanking is a *wrong attitude*. A child should learn from a young age that he is not the center of the universe. A temper tantrum is nothing but a manifestation of a wrong attitude, and should therefore be corrected. And if a child is commanded to do something and he does so unwillingly, fussing or whining, his attitude needs correction too.

Children should be allowed and encouraged to say and ask their parents anything. The boundary is that they do so in a respectful and decent manner. "Mom, I think you are being unfair," would probably be answered with, "Yes, you are right. I am sorry." "You are being so d—n unfair," however, should definitely be corrected.

Last, but definitely not least, discipline is for the *protection* of our children. If a child is doing something that can harm him, a spanking is appropriate. We recently saw a child who had been digging a nail into the flesh of his thumb until the bone became visible. It took a number of spankings to help him get rid of this harmful habit. It is also appropriate to spank a 3-year-old who perches himself on the balcony of a three-story home, like the boy we discussed in chapter four. In fact, if any of our children had done something like this, we would probably have made an exception and spanked him even if we had never given him any instruction in this regard. We do not think it is a viable alternative to wait until he does it a second time and maybe falls off the balcony and fractures his skull. According to the evolutionists, that would be the appropriate thing to do. According to their views, the natural consequences of the child's actions—his fractured skull—would discipline him so that in the future he would be able to apply self-discipline. What a terribly illogical idea and what an irresponsible attitude!

Q *When I command my child to do something, should I always warn him that he will be spanked if he does not obey?*

A If you have never spanked your child or children and have decided to obey God by following this route from now on, the appropriate thing to do would be to arrange a family meeting. Explain to your child or children that God has commanded parents to discipline their children, and specifically to discipline with the rod. During such a family meeting, it would be a good idea to read some appropriate verses from the Bible.

However, if every time you give your child an instruction you add, ". . . otherwise you will be spanked," at the end of the instruction, you are conditioning the child that he only needs to obey commands that are accompanied by threats. At school, he will also only listen to his teacher when threatened, and later in his life only listen to his employer when threatened. Furthermore, it indicates a complete lack of trust in your child. If you give your child an instruction, you should have the trust that he will obey. If he proves himself unworthy of your trust by disobeying, you must spank him, and then trust him again.

In this regard, one should always keep in mind that love evokes love. A parent who loves his child and shows his love, will be loved in return. Likewise, respect evokes respect. The parent who treats his child with respect will command the respect of his child. Hatred and disrespect, on the other hand, evoke hatred and disrespect. The parent who shouts and screams and yells, thereby displaying hatred and disrespect for the child, will be hated in return and will not have the respect of his child. In exactly the same way, trust evokes trust. If you always threaten your child, you will show distrust and then he will not have any trust in you.

Q *Should a parent spank with his or her hand or with some other object, such as a wooden spoon or a belt?*

A A parent's hand is the instrument with which he should express love towards his child—with which he holds, hugs or caresses the child. If one uses one's hand as a spanking tool, there is the very real danger that the child will fear his parent. You do not want your child to flinch every time you put out your hand to touch him, do you? That is why the Bible states that one should use a rod, an *impersonal* object, which has no relation to the parent.

We strongly advise against a wooden spoon, as it is not flexible and could well inflict injury. The purpose of a spanking is not to cause permanent damage, but only to hurt enough so that it can correct a child's behavior or his attitude. A belt is quite acceptable as long as it is held in such a way that it will not curl over to strike the child's hips. His bottom should be used for spanking and no other place on his body.

If you use a belt, it should *not* be one that Dad removes from his waist because it is not impersonal.

The place in the house where the child is spanked should also be the most impersonal room in the house, such as a bathroom. Your child's room is very personal to him, as your room is to you.

Q *Should one remove a child's clothing?*

A Obviously if a child is wearing a thick jacket you will let him take it off. But you certainly don't let him take off his pants. The objective is to correct, not to humiliate.

Q *What is the correct procedure to follow when spanking a child?*

A Just as obedience should be prompt, punishment should also be prompt. Mothers should never use fathers as a threat. Mothers who say, "Wait until your father gets home tonight," teach their children that women have no authority. Their children will certainly not be obedient at school when they have female teachers.

Before a parent spanks his child, he should explain to the child why he (or she) is being punished and what the correct conduct would have been. The focus should be on the folly in the heart of the child, of which the misdeed is a symptom, and not on the child himself. Reproaches such as "Wasn't that an ugly thing to do?" or "How could you have done that?" must be avoided. The folly should be addressed, such as "You have lied and therefore I have to punish you. I punish you so that you can learn to always speak the truth."

After the spanking is over, put the rod (or belt) down, take your child in your arms, and tell him that you love him. Just remember, though, that the bathroom should not be the only place where you tell your child that you love him. Then a child will deliberately misbehave to hear those words and be hugged. Afterwards, the child should be given the opportunity to apologize to the people he may have wronged.

Q *Spanking makes my son more, and not less aggressive. And less than five minutes after a spanking he will repeat the misdeed. What am I doing wrong?*

A You are probably dusting his pants and not spanking him. Although a spanking is not intended to leave any permanent scars, it should still hurt. Without inflicting pain we shall not be able to drive the folly from his heart (see Prov. 22:15). The intention of a spanking is to get the child to repent, and the surest indication that you have accomplished this is genuine tears. There is a huge difference between screaming and yelling, which is a form of resistance against being punished, and genuine tears, which are an expression of remorse. All children show resistance towards punishment. Some scream, some argue, while others wrestle and wriggle.

It is important to note that some children grit their teeth to hold back their tears. This is acceptable behavior. The following idea applies especially to these children, but also to other children. A parent must keep an eye on the long-term results of a spanking. If the child soon commits the same infringement again, it means that the punishment was not severe enough. It is important to keep in mind that the pain thresholds of people differ. What is painful to one child may not be painful to another. Gustav, for example, is easily hurt while Jean is not. He can fall down hard, get up, and continue running. If a child commits the same infringement soon after he has been punished, spank him harder next time. In this way you will find the level where the effect will be of longer duration. The idea is not to spank a child all day and every day, but this is exactly what happens if one merely tickles the child's bottom.

Q *Should the degree of punishment vary according to the degree of disobedience? For example, should I administer three lashes for bullying, five for lying, et cetera?*

A No, besides making the whole issue very complicated, you are missing the point. The aim of biblical spanking is not to avenge the wrong deed or attitude, but to drive folly from the child's heart and bring him to repentance. His misbehavior and wrong attitude are merely symptomatic of the fact that too much folly is still bound up in his heart, in the same way that a cough is a symptom of a cold. Symptomatic treatment is never successful, also in this case. That is why attempts at rehabilitating juvenile delinquents are unsuccessful. Imprisonment avenges the deed, and does not drive folly—the root of the evil—from the juvenile delinquent. Therefore, the aim of spanking should be to drive folly from the child's heart and not to avenge the misbehavior.

Q *Unfortunately, your advice came too late for my 10-year-old son. His behavior problems have accumulated to such an extent through the years that I shall have to spank him morning, noon, and night if I were to correct his behavior. He throws things around when he gets upset (which happens to be very often), constantly bullies his brothers and sisters and our dogs, frequently lies, and cries during homework sessions. Whenever he is corrected he talks back.*

A You are right, you will indeed find yourself doing nothing but spanking your son if you should try to correct all his behavior problems at once. With the aid of a *priority list,* however, you can sort out his problems one by one. The first step would be to compile a list of all the problems that need to be corrected. After all the problems have been listed, the next step would be to prioritize the list. The first one on the list should be the problem that needs to be addressed most urgently, while the last one on the list will be the problem that you feel is least important and can be sorted out at a later stage.

Example of a Priority List:

The priority list below serves as an example only. You should compile your own list.

Priority Number	List of Problems
1.	Throwing things around
2.	Bullying of siblings
3.	Bullying of pets
4.	Back-chatting
5.	Crying during homework sessions
6.	Lying
7.	Swearing

Start working only on the number one problem on your priority list, ignoring all the other problems that appear on the list. Explain to your child that he will not be allowed to throw things around from now on. Also explain to him *why* this kind of behavior is inappropriate. Punish him when he throws something in anger again and every time he throws something after that.

As soon as a whole day has passed without having to punish your child for throwing something, you can start addressing problem number two on the list. Tell your child that he will not be allowed to hit and kick his brothers and sisters from now on.

While working on number two on the list, you will still ignore all items that follow further down the list. You will only punish your child when he bullies his brothers or sisters. Number one on the list, however, should still be maintained. This implies that if your child throws something again, you will immediately punish him for it. As soon as a whole day has passed without having to correct number two on the list, you can start addressing number three. In this way you can work through the whole list of problems, addressing them one by one.

The priority list is not static, meaning that if you only started with three problems on the list, you can later add new problems to the list as may become necessary. You can also, at any time, reprioritize the list, thereby ensuring that you continue addressing the most pressing problems first.

Even though you are addressing his problems one by one, in the initial stages of the process your child will probably have to be punished more often than most other children. This, unfortunately, is unavoidable. The situation can be compared to that of Nur Allah of Sudan, whose problem of malnutrition could only be solved by for some time giving him *more* food than to a normal person. Gradually, your child's behavior will become better and better, and occasions where punishment is required will become fewer and fewer.

Q *What are the causes of bed-wetting, and should one spank a child for it?*

A Little is still known of the causes of bed-wetting. The child who wets his bed is probably not doing so willfully and, therefore, a spanking is not appropriate. One should consider the fact that he is sleeping.

It is accepted that bed-wetting can have three causes. The first is that it is an emotional reaction caused by a lack of security. In the same way that a lack of food can cause a swollen abdomen, a lack of discipline can cause bed-wetting. This is why so many children with ADHD have this problem. In many cases, the bed-wetting stops once the child's need for security has been addressed adequately.

Second, bed-wetting can be or become a habit. Susan's younger son had the problem for a little while: "I was quite certain that the cause was habitual and in order to break the habit, I let him wash his bed-sheets the next morning. I was very careful not to humiliate him. He was already feeling very humiliated by his problem. I said, 'Quickly wash the sheets before anybody else will know you have had an accident.' While he was washing the sheets, I impressed on him that he should get up at night if he felt like going to the toilet. Washing the bed-sheets is not really punishment, but the purpose is to give him something to do that is more unpleasant than having to wake up and get up at night to go to the toilet. In the case of my son, it worked quickly because after washing sheets three mornings in a row, the habit was broken."

Thirdly, bed-wetting can have a physical cause. It may be that the sphincter muscles of the bladder are too weak. The following exercise is usually very effective to correct this.

Let the child sit on a chair. He must now contract the muscles of the anus and try to pull the anus upward. This action simultaneously contracts the sphincter muscles of the bladder, thereby exercising and strengthening them. Let him hold the muscles tight for about ten seconds, and then relax. Let him repeat this sequence of contraction and relaxation ten times every day.

As you do not know exactly what the cause of your child's bed-wetting is, we recommend that you address all of the three probable causes simultaneously. Get your discipline right, break the habit, and do the exercise as described. Also, make sure that he does not drink too much liquid shortly before bedtime.

Q *Until what age is corporal punishment appropriate?*

A Many people have come to believe that spankings should not be given once a child reaches the age of 13. Ideally, a child should not have to be spanked by the time the teenage years are reached.[8] It would be unwise, however, to make a firm rule and say a teenager should never be spanked. Proverbs 19:18 is quite clear in this when it states, "Discipline your son, for in that there is hope; do not be a willing party to his death."

If a child has been trained with the rod of reproof from his early years, the need for spankings will become less and less as the child grows older. The purpose of a spanking in the early years is to help form a child's character in righteousness. Once this character is formed, it will be normal for a child to have good behavior.[9] Yet, he is still a human being and is therefore still fallible.

Susan can still remember her last spanking which was administered by her mother when she was in eleventh grade: "I shall probably never forget this hiding, as it was the most painful one I had ever had. My best friend left school at the end of tenth grade (this was in 1979) and went to a technical college. This meant that she was often at home while I was still in school. I thought this to be unfair and started playing truant to go to her house. I did this more and more often. Later, I did not only skip two or three periods; I stayed away from school the whole day. This continued until my mother caught me red-handed. Oh boy, she really did not tickle my behind that day. She also phoned the school, and the following day the headmaster spanked me on my hands, which was an acceptable way of disciplining girls in those days. Did it work? It must have because I never did it again, and my grades, which were at their lowest at that point, jumped from D's and E's to A's, B's and C's over the next few months. And you know what? I still thank my mom for helping me get on the right track again."

Q *If incorrect behavior and attitudes should be punished, should correct behavior and attitudes be rewarded?*

A We have nothing against rewards as such. Every employee is rewarded with a salary at the end of every month for work completed. It is, however, essential that rewards be given within the frame of discipline. An example of a reward being given outside the frame of discipline is when a child receives an ice cream when he did exceptionally well in a test, but it is ignored if he failed to study for a test. An employee will not get many more salary checks if he does not continue to do his work. He is bound to lose his job. Another example is when a reward is used to *bribe* a child to obey or to show a certain attitude. Obedience and attitudes such as friendliness and honesty cannot be bought, they must be *taught*.

Second, rewards may not be excessive. "I am proud of you" can sometimes be the reward. Third, a child needn't be rewarded for every little thing. The danger is—especially when coupled with excessiveness—that his motivation will later be determined only by external factors, and not by internal factors. He will later do nothing unless there is the external motivation of a reward.

Q *You explained in your book how so-called blind following of authority during World War II was used as a tool to degrade authoritarianism. A gang leader also has "authority," and I certainly would not want my child to follow a gang leader because he has been taught to follow me?*

A Part of your education to your child should be to teach him what true authority is. A "leader" who leads one into doing wrong is not a true leader and is therefore not worthy of being followed. Even a parent who commands a child to do something wrong is not worthy of being followed. Susan got some of this medicine when commanding her elder son to work on a Sunday: " I shall do it tomorrow," he said, "as today is Sunday." He had obviously paid close attention to our discussion of the Ten Commandments some time before.

"I got some more medicine when I recently suggested to my son that he should cut his hair in a certain style because 'everybody else is doing it.' This was a stupid remark, as I constantly warn my sons that something is not necessarily right because 'everybody else is doing it.' His answer certainly took me by surprise: 'So if everybody else uses drugs, is it then okay for me to do it, too?' "

Q *One of my friends allows her young children to watch adult-only videos and read adult-only magazines. Her view is that they will do so behind her back anyway, so she can just as well allow it in her home.*

A One should use a bit of logic here. Why not be consistent and also supply one's children with a variety of drugs, such as heroin and LSD. One can just as well supply them, because that will stop them for using it behind their parents' backs. What is the difference?

We know very well that children sometimes do things that are wrong behind their parents' backs. We were children, too. But the difference is that a child who does something behind their backs *knows* that he is doing something wrong. He has made a *choice* between right and wrong, and he knows very well that he has made the wrong choice. The chance exists that, at some stage, his conscience will get the better of him.

A child, however, who is allowed to do whatever he likes in the presence of his parents, will believe this to be an acceptable way of behavior. How can drugs be wrong if Mom supplies me with it? And how can violence and extramarital sex be wrong if Mom allows my young mind to be filled with violent or perverse images all day?

He simply won't know that it is wrong and his ignorance will influence his behavior for life. In a twenty-two-year study, researchers tracked the development of 875 third graders from a rural community in New York. Among the findings was that those who watched the largest amount of violent television at the age of eight, were the most likely to show aggressive behavior at nineteen and later. About one-quarter of the students were considered violent at thirty—they had been convicted of a crime, had multiple traffic violations or were abusive to spouses."[10] Considering the statistics, that by the age of sixteen the typical American child has been *allowed by their parents* to witness an estimated two hundred thousand acts of violence—including thirty-three thousand murders[11]—it shouldn't surprise anyone that youth violence is on the increase.

Q *You said that parents should not act as friends to their children. Are you suggesting that a parent should not play with his child or children?*

A Of course not. Playing with one's children creates great opportunities for learning, such as being able to adhere to rules, waiting one's turn, and being able to lose. Sometimes learning should not be the objective, but simply having fun with one's child or children. However, the fact that the parent has to lower himself intellectually to adapt to the comprehension or intellectual level of the child in order to fit into his games, should not be seen by the child as a warrant to treat his parent with disrespect or disdain. There is always a line that may not be overstepped, even while playing.

Q *What are the most important ingredients for successful parenthood?*

A *A balanced approach:* There is balance in everything God has made, and a time and a place for everything. A few examples of a balanced approach are as follows: (1) There is nothing wrong with a child who is active and talkative, but he should be taught when and where to sit still and keep quiet; (2) Allow your children to watch TV, but be particular about how much time they spend in front of the television set and about what they watch. Youth violence cannot be blamed on the TV, but on what children are *allowed* to watch by their parents; (3) Give them balanced discipline, i.e. loving discipline.

Sensitivity to the needs of one's children: Although all people have the same needs, every child is unique and different, and the quantity of his needs will differ from that of other children. Some children need more food, more love, more discipline, and more intellectual stimulation than other children. A child who is having difficulties in school, for example, may have a greater intellectual need than most other children.

Stop looking for excuses: Although some children are harder to educate, no child is ineducable. All children can be taught to obey and behave.

Try your best: No parent can be perfect. Parents are human, too. So accept that you *are* going to make mistakes. But fear of erring should not stop one from striving to be the best parent for the child or children God has placed in one's care. Although the responsibility that rests on parents' shoulders is tremendous, the wonderful thing is that He has given us a share in the way our children play their part in the game of life. If God had given us angels, we would have had no share. Then our only role would have been that of an onlooker, watching passively as they grow. But He has given us *children.* Now we can be actively involved, like a potter who is molding a piece of clay on his pottery wheel in order to make a beautiful clay pot.

Trust in God: Trust in God, and not in man. As you have seen, psychology and psychiatry do not have the answers. Only God has all the answers, because He is the origin and source of all wisdom.

Notes

1. Campbell, R., *How to Really Love Your Child,* cited in W. Sears, *Creative Parenting* (Cape Town: Struik Timmins, 1990), 217.

2. Lessing, R., *Spanking: Why, When, How?* (Minneapolis, MN: Bethany House Publishers, 1982), 25.

3. www.crimelibary.com

4. Ibid.

5. Lessing, *Spanking: Why, When, How?,* 35.

6. Ibid., 44.

7. Ibid., 45-46.

8. Ibid., 88-89.

9. Ibid.

10. Toufexis, A., et al., "Behavior: Our violent kids. A rise in brutal crimes by the young shakes the soul of society," *Time,* 12 June 1989, 52+.

11. Ibid.

19.

From Theories to Practice

by Susan du Plessis

His IQ was 148, yet 18-year-old Werner Louw could hardly read. When his reading efficiency was assessed by means of an *ophthalmograph* or *eye-camera* on 9 March 1990—one of the many assessments he had undergone in his life—it was found to be equal to that of a second-grade child. This meant that his reading ability was about ten years behind his chronological age. His eyes fixated 164 times and regressed thirty-six times with every one hundred words of reading. His reading speed was only 107 words per minute (see table on page 283 for more details). It is thus quite understandable that Werner had been battling since his first year in school. He attended third grade in a remedial class for two years, after which he was placed in a school for learning-disabled children, repeating third grade for the third time. His condition was diagnosed as "minimal brain dysfunction." Although his parents went from pillar to post to try and solve his reading problem, nothing seemed to help. As he grew older, a sense of inferiority took hold and he had to receive treatment for depression. "I didn't know what to do, which way to turn. Nothing we did seemed to help his problem," his mother told a reporter.[1] It was thus with great skepticism that the Louw parents came to see Dr. Jan Strydom, a South African educationist and coauthor of this book to try yet another avenue.

Five months later, after working faithfully according to Dr. Strydom's recommendations for two half-hour sessions per day, five days per week, Werner's reading efficiency was retested. It then equaled a ninth-grade level. The number of fixations dropped to 87 and regressions to 3. His reading speed was now 163 words per minute.

Six months after this second reading test, Werner's reading efficiency was tested once again and found to be equal to a second-year college level. His eyes now fixated only 73 times in 100 words. The number of regressions, already low, remained the same. He could now read 230 words per minute. This means that, in less than one year, Werner's reading efficiency level improved by twelve years.

Needless to say, this newly found reading ability changed Werner's life. Today, he is an architect.

The Eye-Camera and Its Application

The eye-camera works as follows: by measuring the time it takes a person to read a piece of text, his *reading speed* per minute is calculated. The movements of the person's eyes are photographed and represented on a reading graph.

This reading graph can be analyzed to determine the number of eye *fixations* that occurred during reading. When a person reads, his eyes engage in a series of quick movements across the page with intermittent fixation pauses. The more often the eyes have to pause for fixations, the slower the reading speed will be. A dyslexic person will be inclined to pause more often, and the duration of each fixation will also be longer than that of the typical reader. After this, it is possible to calculate the person's recognition span. This refers to the average number of words the person can recognize in one fixation, as well as to the average duration of such a fixation.

By analyzing the reading graph one can also determine whether any *regressions* occurred in the eye movements of the reader. A regression occurs when the eyes move toward the left to look again at words that have been covered already. The dyslexic person is inclined to have more regressions than the normal reader.

After reading the piece of text, the person doing the test is required to answer a number of questions on the contents. This is to determine his *comprehension*, which is expressed in a percentage. Lastly, the *relative reading efficiency* can be calculated, which is expressed in year levels.

The test results of Werner are shown on the chart on the following page. The solid line represents the first reading test on 9 March 1990, the thin dashed line the retest on 5 August 1990 and the thick dashed line the second retest on 12 February 1991.

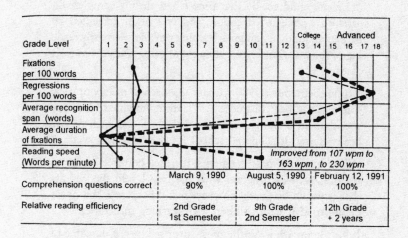

A Program of Hope

The change in Werner's life was brought about by an educational invention of Dr. Strydom, which started life as a school readiness program in the 1970s. The program is named *Audiblox*. *Audi* is derived from "auditory," because the program—among others—enhances auditory skills, while *blox* refers to the main materials used in the program—little colored blocks. The program aims at systematically developing through regular exercise the foundational skills necessary for school and after-school learning—also the foundational skills of reading, discussed in chapter fifteen.

Dr. Strydom believes that the first formative years of a child's life are of the utmost importance. Therefore, he spent a lot of time preparing his own children for formal school learning. However, only when the youngest one was preschool did he hit on the idea of devising a more or less formal school readiness program for her. He continues the story:

> When this daughter entered school, it soon became evident that she was able to learn to read exceptionally quickly and also remarkably well. Soon after school entrance, her teacher remarked that she had never before encountered a child who was so perfectly ready for school as this little one was. From this, I concluded that the program was effective enough to justify making it available to other parents.

At first I recommended the program only to parents with preschool children. By that time I had already completed a master's degree in education, and was often consulted by parents about their children's learning problems—mostly reading problems—but I never thought of using *Audiblox* in such cases.

Late in September 1980 parents approached me about their son who had been diagnosed as "learning disabled." The boy was then in a third-grade remedial class, and had already been referred to a special school for the following year.

While interviewing the parents, the idea occurred to me to try the *Audiblox* program with the boy. I told the parents that it would be purely an experiment, because I had never before tried it with children with learning difficulties.

I don't know who was the most surprised by the outcome of the experiment—the parents or me. Within a mere two months it became quite evident that it would be a grave error to allow this boy to go to a special school. This became apparent not only to his parents and to me, but also to the boy's teacher. She brought this to the attention of the principal of the school, who then called in the school psychologist. After reassessment, it was decided not to send the boy to a special school, but to promote him to the next class the following year.

Later, this boy became a top achiever with marks usually above 80 percent and often above 90 percent. I remember the year he was in seventh grade his father phoned me one evening early in December. They had just returned from the school where their son had been awarded the prize for the top achiever in the school.

This event convinced him that there were far greater possibilities in the *Audiblox* program than he had imagined. Thereafter he started using the program more and more for children with learning difficulties, mostly with resounding success. At first, he used it only for smaller children, but as his confidence grew, he later started to use it for primary school children in the senior classes, still later for high school children, and still later for adults.

Eventually, he adapted his program so that it could also be used in a classroom situation. In this way, not only one at a time, but a whole class full of children could simultaneously benefit from the program. One of the first schools to use the program on a large scale was the Arthur Matthews Primary School in Johannesburg. Every class in the school had one *Audiblox* period per day. Mr. Jan Venter, who has in the meantime retired, was principal of the school. He reported that before he introduced *Audiblox* in his school, he used to require help from the school psychological services for up to 15 percent of his approximately four hundred pupils. After introducing this program, the teachers were able to deal with all but one or two who were in need of individual counseling.[2] Many other mainstream schools have since also introduced this method with great success.

Many years later, with more research and many adjustments to the program, it could also be implemented with great effect for the mentally challenged.

For many years after its initial publication, one question had been plaguing Dr. Strydom. *Why* does a program that he devised for *school readiness* achieve such phenomenal results when used for children with *learning difficulties?* "I always believed that any practice should be supported by a sound theory," he said. "With *Audiblox* I had accidentally stumbled upon a practical method that could achieve wonderful results when used for learning-disabled children, but I had no theoretical explanation for the success of the program. Why was it possible with such a simple program to achieve what learning disabilities experts throughout the whole world had asserted to be impossible—to cure a learning disability? What in *Audiblox* made it possible to help learning-disabled children to become at least normal, often very good, and sometimes even top achievers at school?"

After an intensive study over many years, of the literature on a variety of subjects, including learning and learning disabilities, the answer to this riddle gradually started dawning upon him. I can still remember his excitement when the first two pieces of the puzzle fell into place, i.e., that there is nothing that any human being knows, or can do, that he has not learned, and that human learning is a stratified process. This was in 1988. I had just become involved in the *Audiblox* project and, to be honest, I did not understand his excitement. It is only later that the full significance of this dawned upon me, that if one has a viable point of departure at one's disposal—in this case universal learning principles—one has a firm base on which to build a successful practice. Although a successful practice already existed in the form of *Audiblox,* there was still much room for improvement. And indeed many improvements to the program became possible once we arrived at a better understanding of the idea of foundational skills of learning, reading and writing.

Although repetition was always the backbone of *Audiblox*, the discovery of the third learning principle, that a "pyramid of repetition" must be constructed, added more value to the program. The program was thus changed in accordance with this learning principle. The discovery of this principle also opened new vistas for the mentally challenged. We found that the building blocks of reading and writing, and of learning as such, are the same, whether one is teaching a mentally handicapped or a normal person. The only difference is that these steps have to be broken up into much smaller steps, and these smaller steps have to be repeated many times more before one can move to a following step.

A fact that must be clearly stated is that *Audiblox* is no quick fix for a learning difficulty. It requires hard and diligent work, in most cases preferably by the parents, over a period of time. If the program is stopped before the foundational skills of reading and learning have been *automated*, a relapse will occur.

The Destruction of South Africa's Youth

But, while the program was becoming more and more effective (the latest version of the program is named *Audiblox 2000*), the children of South Africa have at the same time been deteriorating emotionally and intellectually. I have been a witness to a tremendous deterioration in our children since the start of my involvement with *Audiblox* in 1988. The learning difficulties that one encounters today often make those of Werner Louw seem to have been trivial.

One of the more disturbing features of this deterioration is that language problems are on the increase. Since 1988 up to a few years ago, there has always been the odd case of a child whose language ability was not up to standard. At present, cases of children whose language is behind is becoming more and more common. The first time I saw a child who could hardly talk was in 1993. She was severely mentally handicapped. During only the past six months, more than 30 children—all between four and six years of age—who entered Dr. Strydom's office for the first time could hardly talk. In some cases they could not talk at all. Although some of them are mentally challenged, the majority are not. They have simply been neglected—mostly due to ignorance—in their first formative years.

During the first years of my involvement with *Audiblox* by far the majority of children could be helped to overcome their learning problems by means of *Audiblox* group classes, where a general program was followed. Two to three classes per week of one hour each, over a period of eight to twelve months, were usually sufficient to solve their problems. Today, this is no longer the case. The extent of the learning problems that one encounters today has made the group intervention unsuccessful for a great number of children. Many have to be tutored individually and sometimes even their programs have to be *individualized*. Two to three hours per week are often insufficient.

Another change which I have witnessed since 1988 was the increase in the number and severity of behavior problems. In 1988, cases of children with severe behavior problems existed, but were few and far between compared to what one encounters today. I have become accustomed to parents who complain about their children who bully other children, hurt animals, set fires, steal, and are sexually promiscuous at an age when I was still totally ignorant about the subject. In a recent case, the parents of a 7-year-old boy came to see Dr. Strydom because he often exposes his genitals to his classmates, grabs them by their genitals, and often leaves the class for five to ten minutes to masturbate in the toilet. He also has multiple other problems. His parents, unfortunately, refused to accept that a lack of discipline, love, and respect is at the heart of his problem. According to them, they are *too* strict because they constantly shout and scream at the child. They failed to grasp that shouting and screaming is not discipline, but a sign of disrespect and hatred. They are now exploring other avenues.

The most dramatic changes for the worse, however, which I have witnessed over the past few years, were the changes in the attitude of children. In the past, most children needed no or little encouragement to do *Audiblox*. Because the exercises in the program are challenging, most children actually enjoyed them. Those who did not want to do it were seldom given a choice by their parents. They simply had to do it. Their initial stubbornness soon turned to eagerness, because it gradually became possible for them to do the exercises with more and more blocks. Children, who at the start failed to get a sequence of five blocks in the correct order, later managed to do the same exercise with thirty blocks, still later with seventy—a great boost for their self-esteems.

The number of children who enjoy *Audiblox* is becoming smaller and smaller. Very often, those with so-called ADHD actually hate it. When confronted by the mental effort required by the program, many of them cry, or scream, or swear. Others just don't care. The problem is that they are not *emotionally* receptive to learning (see chapter fifteen). This means that they are not willing to learn. The problem is also that, unless they are *made* willing to learn, they cannot be *taught*. This then, is a major reason why children with ADHD have so many academic problems compared to normal children. They have been *allowed* to have a negative attitude toward learning. Often their IQ scores are also lower than those of normal children because of this. One cannot measure a child's true IQ if he is disinterested in any mental effort. An IQ test requires mental effort. The knowledge backlog, caused by their unwillingness to learn over an extended period of time, should of course also be kept in mind. Many of the items used to measure a child's IQ depend on knowledge.

Unfortunately, the *only* method which is successful in correcting a negative attitude—i.e., changing the *heart* of the child—is the rod of reproof. Time-out, taking away privileges, or shouting and screaming will *not* lead to a change of heart. I have seen this time and time again. Parents who are not willing to follow this route have only one option. They will have to accept the label of ADHD and its attending consequences. It is only those parents who are willing to change the hearts of their children who can help their children to overcome their intellectual problems.

It must be stressed again that a child should never be punished for something he cannot do. You cannot punish a child for not being able to read. You can and should, however, punish him for his unwillingness to be taught, for example when he cries, screams, or shows other forms of disinterested or unwilling behavior.

The changing attitudes of South African children are a great source of concern to me, but I am certainly not the only person who has become aware of it. A fifth grade teacher told me that nearly 40 percent of the children in her class are totally disinterested in schoolwork. Some of them are also disruptive, often making it impossible for her to teach those children who *are* emotionally receptive to learning—those who *want* to learn. She blames the chaos in her classroom on the abolition of corporal punishment in 1996. Although she has been in the teaching profession for more than twenty-five years, she has never used the rod herself. The fear of the rod alone used to be sufficient to maintain discipline. "Now my hands are tied," she said. I have no doubt that parental intervention can solve her problem, but at present it seems to make matters worse. "Complaining to the parents about their children's misconduct is mostly a waste of time," she said, "because the parents take sides with their children. The result is that their behavior deteriorates even more. Education has become a 'right,' and is no longer a privilege." She is quitting at the end of the year because she can no longer stomach the disrespect with which she is being treated. "I am scared of some of the children," she said.

To my mind, psychology and psychiatry are the sole culprits for the decay of South Africa's youth. James R. Brown, who has a master's degree in sociology, recently commented about America's youth: "This generation of children is not the product of parental upbringing. This generation, and its destructive behavior, is the direct product of psychology and social work intervention."[3] The same is true of South Africa's children. As nearly everywhere else, one can today hardly open a magazine nor switch on the radio or TV without being bombarded by expert advice. As more expert advice is being published or broadcast, the higher the statistics climb regarding juvenile delinquency, drug abuse, teenage pregnancies, teen suicides, and school failure rates. And the higher the statistics go, the more often the experts are consulted.

If you think that I am being unjustly critical of these two disciplines, the full story is that it had always been my dream to become a psychologist—specifically a *pastoral* psychologist. In order to pursue this "noble" career, I completed a six-year course in theology. In my eagerness to reach my goal, I even shortened this long and drawn-out training by doing the required honors degree in psychology extramurally during the fourth and fifth years of my studies in theology.

I came to love psychology—more than theology—and simply hung on the lips of my lecturers. The only time I was ever confronted by any negative view of psychology was when I had to study Jay E. Adam's book, *Competent to Counsel,* which was a prescribed book in my final year of theology. I instantly dismissed the book as the work of an eccentric extremist, and probably one with a low IQ, too. (I sincerely apologize, Dr. Adams, but I did not know better at the time.)

After this six-year study, when there remained only the required master's degree in psychology between myself and the final realization of my dream, I had to face a problem commonly experienced by students—money. This is how I landed on Dr. Strydom's doorstep. But I was there to stay, because by the time I had the money, I knew that I had wasted six years of my life and a lot of money. I have come to the conclusion that psychology and psychiatry and their followers (by "followers" I mean professionals in other disciplines who have become involved in "mental disorders," such as occupational therapists, pediatricians, and neurologists) are destructive to people in general and to children in particular. I have found the experts to be superior in diagnosing, labeling, and drugging children, but inferior in helping them or changing their behavior. The same applies to so-called pastoral psychology. At first my conclusions were based on subjective observations (few parents who knock on Dr. Strydom's door for help have not been to umpteen "experts"), which were later confirmed by scouring the literature.

Today there are probably many people who will refer to me as narrow-minded, fanatic, eccentric, extremist, or fundamentalist. They can call me whatever they like. I also referred to Dr. Jay E. Adams and people like him in these terms. Now I know better. The scales have fallen from my eyes.

A Case Study

When her baby was eventually born after two unsuccessful inductions on Wednesday, 24 January 1989, Heidi Kennedy was jubilant. Not in her wildest dreams did she foresee that her sweet-looking baby boy would eventually develop a behavior problem so severe that it would cause her marriage to hang by a thread and contribute to the family's financial ruin.

Herman was only four days old when he suffered the first of several tonsil and ear infections. He often had colic at night, after which he usually slept two hours at most. During the daytime, he was always fidgeting and whining. Moreover, he became allergic to dairy products, dust, and animal hair. Although his health problems were eventually solved, the inevitable consequence was that he was lagging behind in several of his developmental milestones. At the age of one, Herman could not sit yet. He only sat for the first time two days after his ears had been drained and temporary tubes had been inserted. At last, at the age of one and a half, he gave his first step. The only milestone that never caused concern at any time was Herman's language ability. In this respect, he was miles ahead of his age group—and still is.

Heidi soon began to sense that everything was not in order. Herman was always on the go. He simply could not settle down. At night all his toys were stacked around him so that he could entertain himself. When losing interest in his toys, he would keep himself busy by undressing and dressing himself ad infinitum—over and over and over. Medical assistance was sought, but Heidi's fears were passed off as those of an overanxious mother.

In 1993 Herman's Namibian parents consulted a pediatrician in Walvis Bay. His diagnosis, after a mere ten minutes, was that Herman was mentally retarded (a rather impulsive diagnosis to make if a child's language is above his age group) and suffered from ADHD. His advice to Herman's parents was that they should accept his intellectual defect as nothing could be done to improve his condition. He prescribed Ritalin and Tofranol.

Herman reacted negatively to Ritalin. An hour after the drug had been administered, says Heidi, "he became like a wild animal and would chatter nonsensically without stopping." Ritalin was stopped and replaced by Mellaril, which made him "zombie-like."

Another pediatrician in Cape Town, South Africa, confirmed the diagnosis of the Namibian pediatrician that Herman was mentally retarded and suffered from ADHD. Ritalin was prescribed once again.

The diagnosis of mental retardation came as a great shock to the Kennedy couple. This diagnosis not only changed their attitude toward him but also the way that they handled him. "If I think back," says Heidi, "we were constantly looking for excuses for Herman's poor behavior. The result was that his behavior deteriorated even more."

Because they believed that they would find better help in Cape Town, the couple moved there in December 1994. In January 1995, a child psychiatrist diagnosed Herman with Tourette's syndrome and prescribed Tofranol and Imipramine.

Tourette Syndrome

Before continuing with Herman's case, let us first discuss "Tourette's syndrome." According to the literature, Tourette's syndrome (TS) is an inherited, neurological disorder, characterized by tics. A tic is defined as a brief, repetitive, purposeless, non-rhythmic, and involuntary movement or sound. Involuntary movements are called "motor tics," while involuntary vocalizations are called "vocal tics" or "phonic tics."

The first symptoms of TS are usually facial tics—commonly eye blinking. However, facial tics can also include nose twitching or grimaces. In time, other motor tics may appear, such as head jerking, neck stretching, foot stamping, or body twisting and bending.[4]

TS sufferers may utter strange and unacceptable sounds, words, or phrases. It is not uncommon for a person with TS to continually clear his or her throat, cough, sniff, grunt, yelp, bark, or shout. People with TS may involuntarily shout obscenities (coprolalia) or constantly repeat the words of other people (echolalia). They may touch other people excessively or repeat actions obsessively and unnecessarily. A few patients with severe TS demonstrate self-harming behaviors such as lip and cheek biting and head-banging against hard objects.[5]

But this is hardly the full picture. Many people with TS experience additional problems, such as

- ADHD.[6]
- Learning disabilities, which include reading, writing, arithmetic, and perceptual difficulties.[7]
- Problems with impulse control, which can result in overly aggressive behaviors or socially inappropriate acts.[8]
- Obsessive-compulsive behavior, where the person feels that something must be done repeatedly, such as hand washing or checking that a door is locked.[9] It may be almost impossible for obsessive-compulsive people to keep a job. People who arrange or rearrange papers on their desks all day long or touch their toes repeatedly are not likely to get much work done. Some TS people never even make it through the front door in the morning. They spend the day taking innumerable showers, or feel compelled to touch and re-touch certain objects in the house a certain number of times before leaving. Some obsessive-compulsive patients have recurrent, protracted thoughts about death or sex that haunt them night and day.[10]
- Social problems: TS children often have problems in school because other children may make fun of them or are even afraid of them. Many simply have no friends. Some miss so much school because of twitching that they don't get a chance to form close relationships. Many are left out of social activities, and tend not to be chosen for team sports, or to be elected as class officers, or asked out on dates.[11]

Depression, embarrassment, and despair are an everyday part of life for these unfortunate people. One sufferer who attempted suicide several times remarked, "I started thinking if I kill myself, maybe it would be better for me, because then I wouldn't have to cope with any of this harassing."[12]

As in the case of ADHD, there are no brain tests or blood tests or any kind of tests that can demonstrate or prove that a person has TS. The diagnosis is made on the basis of the physician's observation and/or the history as reported by observers. As in the case of ADHD, the symptoms of TS often don't appear in the physician's office. One source recommended that parents videotape their child's symptoms to show the physician what the child is doing.[13] And, as in the case of ADHD, medication does not solve the problem. At most, it sidesteps the problem in the short term.

A Personal Experience

The first time I heard about Tourette's syndrome was about five years ago. Because I am accustomed to hearing about new disorders being discovered every now and again, I did not pay much attention to it at first. A few months ago, for example, I heard that there is an "Einstein syndrome" on the loose. People who are highly intelligent but battle to read supposedly suffer from it. Einstein was apparently dyslexic.

About the same time when I first heard of TS, my elder son, who was then four, started to blink his eyes continually. As time went by, the blinking became worse and worse. It hardly ever stopped. I honestly did not know what was wrong and much less what to do. At first I thought that his eye blinking was like a stutter and that he could not help it. (Stammering or stuttering, the subject of Dr. Strydom's doctoral thesis, is truly involuntary.) If it were a true deficit, I would have no problem accepting it. I love my son. Yet, as time went by I started to doubt my assumption and wondered if it wasn't merely a bad habit. I tried to intervene. I ignored it, talked nicely, begged, and offered rewards. Nothing worked. It only seemed to make matters worse. People started to make remarks about it and suggested that I take him for a medical examination.

It was six months after the eye blinking first started that I decided to give it one last try—by correcting this purposeless behavior with the rod. I would feel extremely guilty if it did not work, because it would have meant that I had punished my child for something that he could not help. On the other hand, I would feel much worse if I were to discover one day that I could have done something about it and did not. Weighing the two options, I decided that the former was preferable. I discussed it with my husband, who agreed.

To our surprise the first spanking stopped the eye blinking completely for three hours. The second round stopped it for four months and the third forever. Some years later, he had to get another hiding for sniffing continually and recently for continually / making the funniest noises with his mouth. He would not stop with these actions when only instructed to do so.

It was shortly after the second round with the eye blinking that I started reading up on TS, as this diagnosis was becoming the "in" thing in South Africa. As already mentioned, it is frequently used to label children who do not have any tics at all. It was only then that I realized that Gustav was on his way towards developing true TS.

We became involved in this disorder after the experience with my son. Since then I have spoken to a number of parents who were looking for help for their grown-up children who suffered from true TS. Their main concern was that their children were unemployed because they *did not want to work.*

My son, on the other hand, has an abundance of self-motivation. As stated in the previous chapter, he is almost compulsive in his endeavors to succeed and will not stop trying until he gets something right. This tendency I have also witnessed in a few other children who suffered from true TS, and whose parents were willing to follow the same route that I did. Some would call it a sign of perfectionism, but even if this is so, it is definitely a preferable option to the devastation that awaits the TS sufferer.

To summarize, the tics associated with TS are not involuntary. TS is merely the result of a very bad habit that—of course—gets more and more difficult to control as the person gets older. These habits are nothing but the result of the folly, bound up in the heart of every child. And, if discipline is lacking as well, as it was in the case of Herman, it is the proverbial oil on the fire.

Cured from Tourette's Syndrome

In Cape Town, Herman's behavior was becoming more and more erratic by the day. One moment he was in a deep pit, just to be on top of the world the next moment. It gradually became clear that his milestones were far behind, a fact that became an increasing matter of concern. Besides severe concentration problems, fine and gross motor and visual perception problems, he also had a poor visual memory.

Yet, even with all his multiple problems, the Kennedys felt that their son deserved a chance to lead a normal life. They therefore rejected the recommendation of a child psychiatrist that he should attend a preprimary class at a special school. They enrolled him at a normal preprimary school instead, and in the afternoons carted him to a physiotherapist, an occupational therapist and a remedial teacher. Two months later, however, Herman was suspended from this preprimary school due to uncontrollable behavior. He was then sent to a Montessori preprimary school.

"It is here in Cape Town that we started to isolate ourselves," says Heidi. "Herman's behavior simply did not allow us to have friends."

After he took off three times in public places—once he was found only after a six-hour search—outings had to be shelved too. Herman simply did not have any fear. He would jump off any height without hesitation and therefore had to be watched constantly.

Work obligations forced the Kennedys to return to Namibia in June 1996. By the end of that year, they applied for entrance at a normal school. But Herman, who had looked forward to going to school, was expelled after only three months due to unacceptable behavior. His sometimes bizarre behavior is summarized by a psychological report, dated 7 March 1997:

- Herman is still impulsive and aggressive. When he passes other children he hits them for no reason. He bit a classmate's finger off. According to his teacher this was an impulsive act.
- He bites his fingernails as well as his toenails.
- He steals continually.
- He has an obsession about paper. He also steals paper. He eats paper compulsively. A classmate was very upset last week when Herman ate his whole birthday card.
- Herman also eats chalk compulsively.
- He swears continually.
- Motor tics: Herman's big toe is moving up and down the whole time. This tic is not absent for a moment.
- Herman is still unable to concentrate, does not sit still, does not listen and does not pay attention.

The psychologist found Herman's IQ to be seventy, which meant that he was "functioning intellectually on a much lower level than other 8-year-olds." Her conclusion was that Herman does not have adequate intellectual, emotional, and social skills to function in mainstream, and recommended a special school where his emotional, social, behavior, and intellectual deficits could be accommodated. Because Namibia did not have such a facility, he would have to go to a special school in South Africa.

The recurring failures on social level caused Herman to be depressed and suicidal thoughts and talk started to develop. He wet his bed several times every night. In August 1997, his by now desperate parents took him to yet another South African specialist. Herman's medication was modified, and when this had no effect, it was modified again and again and again.

By this time, the Kennedy couple's marriage was on the edge of the precipice. Besides Herman being a constant stress factor, the family was ruined financially. Mr. Kennedy had been cheated by his partner and Herman's astronomical medical costs were the last straw.

Most parents would have thrown in the towel by now. Heidi refused. The result of her determination was that Herman passed first grade in 1998 and second grade in 1999—in a mainstream school. The latter he did with flying colors. In his last report he was also praised for his good behavior in class.

An improvement was also noted in his Herman's IQ score. As stated, he scored seventy on 7 March 1997. When his IQ was reassessed in November 1998, it was 84. On 13 June 1999, it was found to be 96. Of course *Audiblox*—which his mother is still doing diligently—contributed to Herman's academic progress. But there is no doubt in my mind that absolutely nothing would have happened on an academic level if his parents were not willing to follow God's instructions. It is *only* their obedience to God that could cause the symptoms of ADHD and TS to disappear. It is *only* their obedience to God that could turn their aggressive and destructive child into a loving child. He is still very active and a real chatterbox, but can now sit still and be dead quiet in situations where it is required of him. He can even be trusted to behave when left on his own. He now goes to bed at eight, after watching one or two programs on TV—something he never did. The obsessive-compulsive behavior, the continual swearing and stealing are things of the past. The bed-wetting gradually diminished and is now nonexistent. Suicidal thoughts and talk no longer occur. The last-mentioned problem was the first to disappear, which convinced Heidi that she was now on the right track. In fact, she was so convinced that she moved again.

Although long-distance training on *Audiblox* is available, she moved to be close to Dr. Strydom's office. Her husband joined them a few months later.

If you think that this is an easy road to walk, be warned that it is not. In Herman's case it was particularly difficult because the discipline situation had been severely neglected for such a long time. When his parents started to intervene in October 1997 according to the recommendations in this book, Herman's priority list looked like a scroll. Twice, after it started looking as if nearly all his problems had been sorted out, he offered stubborn resistance to change, his behavior deteriorating again to such an extent that his parents basically had to start from scratch. But they stuck to what they by then knew was right and are now finally cashing in. And so is Herman, who is on his way toward becoming a success in life.

Besides being a difficult road, it is a lonely road as well. There was a time when the whole community supported and even helped parents to raise their children to become decent adults. That time, unfortunately, belongs to the past. Parents who desire to raise their children to become decent adults are seldom praised. But don't let it stop you. There are many critics and meddlers in the world who are unable to raise a child successfully. God did not choose any of them to raise your child or children. He has chosen *you!* The responsibility, therefore, is *yours,* not theirs.

Notes

1. Kelly, D., "Overcoming dyslexia," *The Citizen,* 24 April 1991, 21.

2. Bassett, H., "Dyslexia: New therapy, new hope," *Fair Lady,* 12 August 1992, 130-132.

3. Brown, J. R., "Warning signs were there," *The New Australian,* no. 118, 10-16 May 1999.

4. "What is Tourette syndrome?" National Institute of Neurological Disorders and Stroke, 1998, website.

5. Ibid.

6. Ibid.

7. Ibid.

8. Ibid.

9. Ibid.

10. Zamula, E., "Taming Tourette's tics & twitches," *FDA Consumer*, vol. 22, 1988, 26-30.

11. Ibid.

12. Gross, T., "Twitch and shout," *Fresh Air (NPR)*, 6 May 1998.

13. "Frequently asked questions," Tourette Syndrome Association, Inc., website.

We welcome comments from our readers. Feel free to write to us at the following address:

Editorial Department
Huntington House Publishers
P.O. Box 53788
Lafayette, LA 70505

or visit our website at:

www.huntingtonhousebooks.com

═══════════

More Good Books from Huntington House Publishers

ABCs of Globalism
A Vigilant Christians Glossary
by Debra Rae

Do you know what organizations are working together to form a new world order? Unlike any book on today's market, the *ABCs of Globalism* is a single volume reference that belongs in every concerned Christian's home. It allows easy access to over one hundred entries spanning a number or fields—religious, economic, educational, environmental, and more. Each item features an up-to-date overview, coupled with a Biblical perspective.

ISBN 1-56384-140-1

Government by Political Spin
by David J. Turell, M.D.

Political Spin has been raised to a fine art in this country. These highly paid "spin doctors" use sound bites and ambiguous rhetoric to, at best, influence opinions, and at worst, completely mislead the public. *Government by Political Spin* clearly describes the giant PR program used by Washington officials to control the information to American citizens and maintain themselves in power.

ISBN 1-56384-172-X

The Deadly Deception
Freemasonry Exposed..
By One of It's Top Leaders
by Jim Shaw and Tom McKenny

This is the story of one man's climb to the top, the top of the "Masonic mountain." A climb that uncovered many "secrets" enveloping the popular fraternal order of Freemasonry. Shaw brings to life the truth about Freemasonry, both good and bad, and for the first ever, reveals the secretive Thirty-Third Degree initiation

ISBN 0-910311-54-4

The Hidden Dangers of the Rainbow
by Constance Cumbey

This nationwide best-seller paved the way for all other books on the subject of the New Age movement. Constance Cumbey's book reflects years of in-depth and extensive research. She clearly demonstrates the movement's supreme purpose: to subvert our Judeo-Christian foundation and create a one-world order through a complex network of occult organizations. Cumbey details how these various organizations are linked together by common mystical experiences. The author discloses who and where the leaders of this movement are and discusses their secret agenda to destroy our way of life.

ISBN 0-910311-03-X

The Coming Collision
Global Law vs. U.S. Liberties
by James L. Hirsen, Ph.D.

Are Americans' rights being abolished by International Bureaucrats? Global activists have wholeheartedly embraced environmental extremism, international governance, radical feminism, and New Age mysticism with the intention of spreading their philosophies worldwide by using the powerful weight of international law. Noted international and constitutional attorney James L. Hirsen says that a small group of international bureaucrats are devising and implementing a system of world governance that is beginning to adversely and irrevocably affect the lives of everyday Americans.

Paperback ISBN 1-56384-157-6
Hardcover ISBN 1-56384-163-0

Cloning of the American Mind
Eradicating Morality Through Education
by B. K. Eakman

Two-thirds of Americans don't care about honor and integrity in the White House. Why? What does Clinton's hair-splitting definitions have to do with the education establishment? Have we become a nation that can no longer judge between right and wrong?

"Parents who do not realize what a propaganda apparatus the public schools have become should read Cloning of the American Mind *by B. K. Eakman."*

—Thomas Sowell, *New York Post*
September 4, 1998

ISBN 1-56384-147-9

The 3 Loves of Charlie Delaney
by Joey W. Kiser

A delightful story of first love, innocence, heartbreak, and redemption. Kiser uses his pen to charm and enchant but most of all...to remind.

ISBN 0-933451-45-8

How to Avoid High Tech Stress
by Robert J. du Puis, M.D.

Technology has created "Instruments of Urgency." such as E-mail, fax machines, cellular phones and pagers, which allow instant communication and transfer of information. It also allows instant accessibility unknown in the past. *How to Avoid High Tech Stress* examines how this instant accessibility has caused increasing levels of stress—instead of freeing us from drudgery.

ISBN 1-56384-159-2

Hormonal Imbalance
The Madness and the Message
by Terry Dorian, Ph.D.

Safe, natural, and effective solutions to problems caused by hormonal imbalance. Discover how to end menopausal symptoms such as stress, confusion, hot flashes, night sweats, etc. Women from the beginning of puberty and throughout the post-menopausal years need this information in order to escape the horrors of hormonal imbalance.

Discover:

- *The deception of conventional Estrogen Replacement Therapy (ERT) and Hormone Replacement Therapy (HRT).*
- *How to end menopausal symptoms (hot flashes, night sweats, vaginal pain, bloating, and more) and reverse aging.*
- *Why you don't have to suffer from PMS.*
- *How to prevent and reverse osteoporosis, heart disease, and memory loss.*
- *Who the healthiest people in the world really are and why.*

ISBN 1-56384-156-8

Liberalism
Fatal Consequences
by W. A. Borst, Ph.D.

Liberalism indicted! *Liberalism: Fatal Consequences* will arm conservatives of all kinds (Christians, Orthodox Jews, patriots, concerned citizens) with the necessary historical and intellectual ammunition to fight the culture war on any front as it exposes the hypocrisy of liberalism.

"...an excellent critical examination of the issues that threaten to divide our nation."

—President Roche, Hillsdale College

ISBN 1-56384-153-3